Promoting Health
A Practical Guide to
Health Education

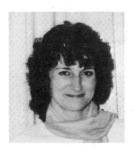

Linda Ewles *MSc BSc SRD*

Linda Ewles is District Health Education Officer for Bristol and Weston Health Authority. After working for a number of years in hospital and community dietetics in England and Bermuda, and as a health education officer in East Sussex, she was Senior Lecturer in Health Education at Bristol Polytechnic for several years. This involved teaching health education, nutrition and communication to students on health visiting, district nursing, community psychiatric and mental handicap nursing and nursing degree courses. She also directed the post-graduate Diploma in Health Education, the recognized qualification for health education officers.

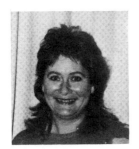

Ina Simnett *MA(Oxon) DPhil CertEd*

Ina Simnett is a Training Consultant with the National Health Service Training Authority at their Headquarters in Bristol. She started her career as a research physiologist, then worked as an adult education tutor and freelance broadcaster while bringing up her three daughters. Following teacher training and a period as a biology teacher and sixth-form tutor, she worked in health education for twelve years as Area Health Education Officer for Northumberland Health Area and a period as a Regional Coordinator for the Health Education Council ''Understanding Alcohol'' programme in South-west England. She has extensive experience of teaching health education to health professionals, teachers and social services staff. She is co-author of a training manual for alcohol educators, and is one of a team disseminating a national programme of training key tutors in alcohol education.

Both authors' activities include presentations at national and international conferences, and serving on national professional associations and advisory bodies on health education.

Promoting Health

A Practical Guide to Health Education

Linda Ewles MSc BSc SRD

Ina Simnett MA(Oxon) DPhil CertEd

An H M + M Publication

JOHN WILEY & SONS
Chichester · New York · Brisbane · Toronto · Singapore

H M+M Publications is an imprint of John Wiley & Sons Ltd

Library of Congress Cataloging in Publication Data:

Ewles, Linda.
  Promoting health, a practical guide to health
education.

  (A Wiley medical publication)
  Includes bibliographies and index.
  1. Health education. 2. Mass Media in health education.
3. Medical personnel and patient. I. Simnett, Ina.
II. Title, III. [DNLM: 1. Health Education.
2. Health Promotion. QT 200 E95P]
RA440.5.E94 1985   613'.07   84-29095
ISBN 0 471 90514 3

British Library Cataloguing in Publication Data:

Ewles, Linda
  Promoting health: a practical guide to health
  education.
  1. Health education—Great Britain
  I. Title   II. Simnett, Ina
  613'.07'041   RA440.3.G7

  ISBN 0 471 90514 3

Phototypeset by Dobbie Typesetting Service, Plymouth, Devon
Printed by Page Brothers, Norwich, Norfolk

Preface

The aim of this book is to provide an easy-to-read, practical guide for health professionals and others who practise health education as part of their everyday work. The health professionals we refer to include hospital and community nurses, health visitors, environmental health officers, hospital doctors, general practitioners, dentists, dental therapists and hygienists, midwives, dietitians and chiropodists; teachers, social workers, youth workers and those involved with Youth Training Schemes may also find it useful. For all these people, whether they are students in basic or post-basic training, or qualified professionals with years of experience wishing to take another look at the health education aspects of their work, this book will encourage the establishment of sound principles on which to base their own practice and to develop their skills in a variety of health education methods.

The book is designed to be used as a self-teaching aid and as a source of material and ideas for group teaching by course tutors. We have included exercises, study questions, case-studies, quizzes and cartoons to make learning stimulating, relevant and enjoyable.

The need for a book of this nature has been expressed by tutors and students on Health Education Certificate courses, and by many other health professionals, for three main reasons. One is that health education is an emerging field of study rather than an established discipline in its own right. As a result, it is difficult for the health professional to locate relevant and understandable material, which is scattered throughout a wide range of sources. Secondly, health education is receiving greater emphasis in the training and practice of health professionals. Thirdly, the general public is becoming increasingly interested in health issues, and is expressing a wish for more health education.

We hope that this book will challenge, inform and help to develop the professional practice of health education.

LINDA EWLES
INA SIMNETT
January 1985

Contents

Acknowledgements

We are indebted to numerous people who have shared with us their health education experience and ideas. They include members of courses such as Health Education Diploma and Certificate courses, basic training courses for a range of health professionals, and professional development courses for teachers, youth workers, social services staff, health workers and others. The exercises contained in the book have been tested with one or more of these groups of students, and without their involvement it would have been impossible to produce a book which is, hopefully, relevant to the real needs and concerns of all health educators and their clients.

We would also like to acknowledge the contribution of all those people who have influenced the development of our own learning and ideas. Special thanks are due to Stella Mountford, Keith Hazeltine, Alan Beattie, Sue Habeshaw, Trevor Habeshaw, John Heron, Donna Brandes, Martin Evans and all the Health Education Officers in the North East.

We are grateful to many people for giving us ideas for exercises included in this book, but especially to Sue Habeshaw and Penny Mares.

We would like to thank Hazel Slavin, Iain Harkess, Jane Randell, George Laidler, Sheila Davison, Michael Whitfield, Margaret Edwards, Noreen Hunt, Heather Ashby and Roger Cartwright for reading draft chapters and offering support and critical comment.

We appreciate the help of Stewart Greenwell with Chapter 14 *Working Collectively*, and Roger Silver with Chapter 15 *Working with the Mass Media*.

Our thanks, too, to Christopher Flook and Christine Flook for drawing the cartoons, and to Adrian Shaw for technical help with the illustrations. We are also grateful to Sue Kennett for patiently typing the final manuscript.

Finally, for their practical and moral support, we thank Patrick West, Jane Randell and Jack Humphreys.

LE
IS

Note on Terminology

We have frequently referred to the health educator as "she", and to the recipient of the health education as "he". This is not, of course, intended to imply that all health educators are female (although many are), nor that people receiving health education are always male. It is simply to avoid confusion and clumsy repetition of "he/she" and "himself/herself".

Also, we have referred to the person receiving the health education as the "patient", the "consumer" or the "client". Where the point being made is likely to be particularly relevant to sick people, we have used "patient"; in other places, we have used "consumer" or "client". This does not imply that where we have referred to patients the text is irrelevant to healthy clients or vice-versa. It is solely to avoid the use of awkward terms such as "patient or client".

Introduction

All health professionals who work with the public will, as part of their everyday work, teach, inform, advise and counsel their clients, individually or in groups. In this way, all health professionals are health educators, although they may not separate this element from the rest of their work (such as treatment, therapy and patient care) and label it "health education". It is evident that by words and example, either deliberately or unconsciously, all health professionals are involved in health education. This book is concerned with the health education aspects of a health professional's job.

We are concerned with the *what, why, who* and *how* of health education itself, as a process carried out by health professionals. We aim to raise and discuss the key questions of

—what do we mean by the term "health education"?
—is it an important activity for health professionals? If so, why?
—what does health education aim to do?
—whose job is it? Who are the agents and agencies of health education?
—who are the consumers of health education?
—how can health education policies and plans be made? How can priorities be set?
—how can health professionals best carry out health education? What are the opportunities, methods, media, strategies, skills and resources required?
—how can the effectiveness of health education be assessed?

These are the fundamental questions we ask readers to consider.

The range of health "topics" is clearly enormous, and health professionals have their own areas of expert knowledge in, for example, child care, nutrition or stress management. Many of these areas of health knowledge will be referred to in this book when we give examples of health education practice but it is not our aim to discuss the *content* of health messages.

We have organised the book into three sections. *Part I Philosophy* deals with basic ideas of what health and health education are about, and the different approaches and ethical issues which need to be considered. *Part II Planning* looks at who does health education, how they decide on needs and priorities, and how they plan their work. *Part III Practice* starts by considering how health educators relate to clients. It then looks at how health educators can develop their skills in a range of health education methods, including teaching, group work, working with the mass media and working collectively with groups of other people.

In this book, we ask the health professional to assess, or reassess, her knowledge, attitudes and values about health and education, her attitude to her clients and her role as a health educator. She needs to establish her own well-reasoned philosophy of health education which she can then incorporate into her professional practice. Unless the health professional sorts her own views out first, she is in no position to help her clients to sort out theirs, or to develop her own skills on a sound basis.

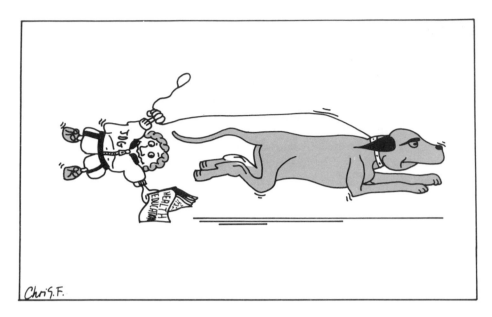

Studying this book will be an active educational experience!

We aim to keep the reader involved, so that studying this book will be an active educational experience. For this reason, we have included exercises for the reader to do as an individual or in a group, and examples and case studies which we hope will help the reader actively to apply ideas to her own situation. Often the exercises are designed to stimulate thought and discussion, and as there may be no "right" answers, we do not provide them. Some readers may find this frustrating, unusual or uncomfortable, because they will find themselves in a state of uncertainty over whether their answers are acceptable or "right". Our response to that is to ask readers to think it through, talk it over and work it out for themselves. In this way, the uncomfortable stage will be worked through and the "answers" will have a personal meaning and application. This is a far more enriching educational experience than the passive absorption of someone else's views.

Health education can best be considered as an applied field of study, which takes knowledge and ideas from other areas and applies them to the specific field of health education. We have identified the following as the main areas from which we draw our material: *health sciences*, particularly epidemiology and environmental health, *social sciences*, notably sociology and psychology, and *education and communication studies*, which in themselves draw upon sociology, psychology and social psychology. We have also drawn on research reports and original journal articles. Of equal importance, we have drawn on our own experience, and that of our colleagues and students.

PART I

PHILOSOPHY

Chapter 1
Concepts and Determinants of Health

Summary

In this chapter the reader is asked to identify which aspects of "being healthy" are the most important to her, and then to examine some lay and professional concepts of health. Physical, mental, emotional, social, spiritual and societal aspects of health are identified. A holistic approach is discussed, followed by an exercise which asks the reader to examine further her own concept of health. This leads into an exercise in analysing the factors which influence health, a review of major areas of current debate about the relative importance of different factors, and a case study. Turning to the question of why put resources into health education, three basic reasons are suggested, followed by illustrative "success stories". Finally, through an exercise and case studies, the reader is invited to develop a personal rationale for her own health education work.

What does Being Healthy mean to You?

"Being healthy" means different things to different people. Much has been written about the concepts of health, and references are given at the end of this chapter for the interested reader.[1] More important than academic discussion, though, is the need for each health professional to explore and define for herself her own concept of health, and what being healthy means to her and to her clients.

Exercise — What does being healthy mean to you?

In Column 1, tick any of the statements which seem to you to be important aspects of your health.

continued on next page

continued

For me, being healthy involves:	Column 1	Column 2	Column 3
1 Enjoying being with my family and friends	_____	_____	_____
2 Living to a ripe old age	_____	_____	_____
3 Feeling happy most of the time	_____	_____	_____
4 Being able to run when I need to (eg. for a bus) without getting out of breath	_____	_____	_____
5 Having a job	_____	_____	_____
6 Being able to get down to making decisions	_____	_____	_____
7 Hardly ever taking tablets or medicines	_____	_____	_____
8 Being the ideal weight for my height	_____	_____	_____
9 Taking part in lots of sport	_____	_____	_____
10 Feeling at peace with myself	_____	_____	_____
11 Never smoking	_____	_____	_____
12 Having clear skin, bright eyes and shiny hair	_____	_____	_____
13 Never suffering from anything more serious than a mild cold, flu or stomach upset	_____	_____	_____
14 Not getting things confused or out of proportion — assessing situations realistically	_____	_____	_____
15 Being able to adapt easily to changes in my life such as moving house, changing jobs or getting married	_____	_____	_____
16 Feeling glad to be alive	_____	_____	_____
17 Drinking only moderate amounts of alcohol or none at all	_____	_____	_____
18 Enjoying my work without much stress or strain	_____	_____	_____
19 Having all the parts of my body in good working condition	_____	_____	_____
20 Getting on well with other people most of the time	_____	_____	_____
21 Eating the "right" foods	_____	_____	_____
22 Enjoying some form of relaxation/recreation	_____	_____	_____
23 Hardly ever going to the doctor	_____	_____	_____

In Column 2, tick the six statements which are the *most important* aspects of being healthy to you.
In Column 3, rank these six in order of importance — put "1" by the most important, "2" by the next most important and so on down to "6".
If you are working in a group, compare your list with other people's.[2]

Lay and Professional Concepts of Health

To the lay public, being healthy may just mean "not being ill". Health is an abstract idea, only given consideration in a negative way when people are thinking about illness or health problems.[3]

There are, perhaps, two other ways in which the general public thinks of health. The first is reflected in phrases like "building up strength" and having "resistance" to infection. This implies that health means strength and robustness, and having reserves which can be called on to fight illness and cope with stress and fatigue. Secondly, people talk about being "off-colour" or "out of sorts" or, conversely, being "in good form". In this way, health may be closely associated with moods and feelings, and a sense of balance and equilibrium.[4]

Standards of what may be considered "healthy" also vary. An elderly person may say she is in good health on a day when her chronic bronchitis and arthritis have eased up enough to enable her to hobble down to the shops. A smoker may not report his early-morning cough as a symptom of ill-health, because to him, of course, it is "normal". People assess their own health subjectively, and this is one of the reasons why attempts to measure health (as opposed to measuring illness) are especially difficult.[5]

To professionals in the health field, "health" may be viewed more objectively as freedom from medically-defined disease and disability. But there may be a world of difference between a lay and professional person's perception of what "counts" as illness or disability.[6]

Several decades ago, the World Health Organisation defined health as "a state of complete physical, mental and social well-being, rather than solely as an absence of disease".[7] This much-quoted statement has subsequently been criticised, mainly on two grounds. One is that it is unrealistically Utopian (how often does anyone truly feel in a state of "complete . . . well-being"?). The other criticism is that it implies a static position, whereas life and living are anything but static. The idea that health means having the ability to adapt continually to constantly changing demands, expectations and stimuli is seen to be preferable.

Towards a Holistic Concept of Health

The exercise *What does being healthy mean to you?* involves the reader in identifying a number of different dimensions in the concept of health. These may be classified as follows.

Physical Health

This is, perhaps, the most obvious dimension of health, and is concerned with the mechanistic functioning of the body.

Mental Health

By mental health we mean the ability to think clearly and coherently. We distinguish this from emotional and social health, although there is a close association between the three.

Emotional Health

This means the ability to recognize emotions such as fear, joy, grief and anger and to express such emotions appropriately. Emotional or "affective" health also means coping with stress, tension, depression and anxiety.

Social Health

Social health means the ability to make and maintain relationships with other people.

Spiritual Health

This, for some people, is connected with religious beliefs and practices; for other people it is to do with personal creeds, principles of behaviour and ways of achieving peace of mind.

Societal Health

So far, we have considered health at the level of the individual. But a person's health is inextricably related to everything surrounding that person and it is impossible to be healthy in a "sick" society which does not provide the resources for basic physical and emotional needs. For example, people cannot be healthy in famine areas, countries of extreme political oppression and, arguably, countries where there is a continual threat of nuclear war. Women cannot be healthy when their contribution to society is undervalued, and neither black nor white can be healthy in a racist society. Unemployed people cannot be healthy in a society which only values people who work, and it is very unlikely that anyone can be healthy living in an area lacking basic services and facilities such as health care, transport and recreation. Michael Wilson[8] graphically says that health cannot be possessed. "It can only be shared. There is no health for me without my brother. There is no health for Britain without Bangladesh."

The identification of these different aspects of health is a useful exercise in raising awareness of just what a complex concept "health" is. But in practice, it is obvious that dividing people's lives into "physical", "mental" and so on often imposes artificial divisions and unhelpful distortions of a situation. All aspects of health are interrelated and interdependent, and we subscribe to the view that a holistic view of health is of greater value to the health professional and her client.

Case study — Dimensions of health

Bob has chronic bronchitis and smokes 20 cigarettes a day. He knows that smoking causes him to cough in the mornings and aggravates his bronchitis. He continues to smoke because it is the only way he can find to cope with the demands of his work. When he tries to stop smoking he feels so tense and irritable that his work suffers and he becomes very bad-tempered with his wife and child. For Bob, his emotional and social health depend on his smoking, and this outweighs the disadvantages to his physical health.

Exercise — Dimensions of health

1. Go back to your answers in the previous exercise *"What does being healthy mean to you?"*
    Which of the following dimensions of health are reflected in the statements you ticked in Column 1:

    physical   _____
    mental   _____
    social   _____
    emotional   _____
    spiritual   _____
    societal   _____

    Which of these dimensions are the most important to you?
    In what ways do the different dimensions relate to each other?
2. Has your idea of "health" changed since childhood? If so, how and why?
    What difference has your professional training made to your idea of health?
3. What do you think "being healthy" may mean to someone who:
    — is mentally handicapped?
    — has a permanent physical disability (eg. is confined to a wheelchair or is deaf)?
    — has a chronic illness (eg. diabetes, arthritis, or a recurring mental disorder such as schizophrenia)?
    — lives on the poverty line in a "third world" country?
4. Identify three or four key points you have learnt from this exercise about your own ideas of "being healthy".

What Affects Health?

Being healthy is rarely, if ever, the result of chance or luck. A state of health or ill-health is the result of a combination of factors having a particular effect on a particular individual at any one time. In order to educate towards better health, it is necessary to identify these influential factors. We suggest that health professionals begin by looking at factors which influence their own health. This is the aim of the exercise overleaf.

There has been much debate in the last decade or so about the relative importance of various determinants of health. In particular, there has been an increasing awareness that medicine, as a professional practice, has had surprisingly, and disappointingly, little effect on people's health. This realization has come about with the knowledge that the introduction of the National Health Service has not, as originally hoped, led to a marked increase in the health of the nation.

Some people have taken this argument further and claim that the practice of Western medicine has, in fact, done considerable harm. The side-effects of treatment, the complications which set in after surgery, and dependence on prescribed drugs are all examples of this. But more important, perhaps, is that control over health and

Exercise — What affects your health?

The aim of this radiating circle exercise is to identify factors which affect your health. The exercise can be done
— individually
— individually, followed by comparing results with other people
— as a group, pooling your ideas about what influences your health.

You are at the centre of the rings:
In the inner ring, write in factors which influence your health *which are to do with yourself as an individual.*
In the second ring, write in factors which influence health *which are to do with your immediate social and physical environment.*
In the outer ring, write in factors which influence your health *which are to do with your wider social, physical or political environment.*

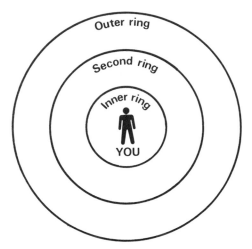

How do these factors influence your health — positively or negatively?
Which factors do you think are the most important?
Are there factors which you have not identified for yourself, but which may be important for other people?[9]

illness has been taken from people themselves, who become dependent on doctors and medicines, expecting a cure for every ill and losing their own ability to cope with sickness, disability and death. Aspects of life which may be difficult, such as adolescence, pregnancy and old age, have been increasingly labelled "medical", and the onus of responsibility shifted from the lay public to the medical profession.

A second area of recent debate and interest concerns the inequalities in health status of different groups of people. It is apparent that, for almost every kind of illness and disability, people in the upper socio-economic classes have a greater chance of avoiding illness and staying healthy than those in the lower classes. There are also differences in the risks to men compared with those to women, and variations in the apparent "healthiness" of living in different parts of the UK. This points to the fact that major determinants of health are concerned with social class, occupation, economic conditions, geographical location and gender.[10]

There is very little, if anything, that individuals can do to change any of these determinants, and this brings us to the third area of debate: the role of individuals in shaping their own health destiny. Some things *can* be done by individuals — more exercise, less smoking, and so on — but these individual changes need to be seen in the context of wider socio-economic situations.

Further reading on determinants of health is given at the end of this chapter.[11] Health professionals need to be aware of the whole range of factors which influence the health of themselves and their clients.

Case study — Determinants of health

Wendy describes her situation this way:
"The most influential people in my life are my husband and my children. My husband supports me financially and provides a good secure home for me and the children. On the negative side, I feel that I'm too dependent on him and have no independent existance outside the home. I am jealous of his involvement in his work and get very anxious when he doesn't get home on time. The children are marvellous — they give me lots of affection — but I get fed up with always having to be on tap to meet their demands.

"Then there's my mother — even though I only see her once a week, she's a strong influence on me. She's always wanting to do things for me — nothing is ever too much trouble — but this leaves me with the feeling that I'm still a child. I would like to get a job or study for a career, but there's no jobs to be had round here and in any case my husband and mother wouldn't approve of me having a job while the children are still small.

"I bottle up my feelings of resentment, and if I'm really honest I suppose I make a martyr of myself.

"I'm overweight and I have secret binges when I just stuff myself with sweets, cakes, chocolate biscuits and sometimes sherry and martini as well. Of course I'd like to be slim but I just can't help myself.

"Recently I haven't been able to sleep properly and the doctor put me on tranquillisers. They don't seem to help much. I feel as if I'm not coping as well as I was before.

"I would like to get out more, but somehow I just can't get myself together.

"I would like to say 'no' to my mum sometimes and not get angry with her."

Wendy identifies the following positive influences on her health:
— good secure home;
— financial support from her husband;
— affection from her children.

continued on next page

continued

She identifies the following negative influences:
— no jobs available;
— demanding relationship with children;
— dependent relationship with husband and mother;
— attitude of husband and mother towards working outside the home.

The results of these influences are:
— no independent existence outside the home;
— inability to take control, say what she wants and change things;
— negative emotions: anxiety, jealousy, resentment and anger;
— unhealthy behaviours: eating binges, secret drinking, sleeplessness and taking tranquillisers.

These influences, and their consequences for Wendy, reflect the values and attitudes of the society she lives in: they include:
— the expectation that women are carers (a woman's place is in the home) which leads to the expectation that Wendy will stay at home, and to her mother's need to have Wendy to care for;
— the expectation that people should bottle up emotions (stiff upper lip), and that women should not assert themselves when it comes to fulfilling their own needs and wants (little girls should be seen and not heard);
— political policies which could be responsible for the lack of available jobs and opportunities for further education and training;
— the attitude of Wendy and her doctor (a pill for every ill). They fail to look at the root causes of Wendy's ill-health and merely attempt to treat the symptoms with tranquillisers. They are unaware that health education about skills in coping, managing negative emotions and assertiveness could help Wendy.

Taking a longer-term view, a combination of political change, education for self-awareness and personal development, and a reduction in sexual inequality could prevent many more people like Wendy ending up in this unhealthy situation.

The "Wendy" case-study has begun to address the question of *why* health education? Why spend time, energy and money educating people about health?

Basic Reasons for Health Education

It is important for each health professional to think through her answer to the question "Why do health education?" The fact that health education is written into her job description, and is part of the policy of her manager, will not be enough to keep her going when things get tough. She needs to be very sure in her own mind about why she thinks health education is an important and valued aspect of her work. She may also need sound reasons to back up a case for the resources to do the job.

Health Knowledge is a Basic Human Right

There is a vast body of knowledge about the factors which influence health for good or ill—knowledge which has the potential to affect the health of every human being.

People have a basic human right to health knowledge, in the same way as they have a right to vote and to have the protection of the law.[12] Giving people health knowledge is a fundamental part of health education.

In most cases, people also *want* to have this health knowledge. This may not be true in certain circumstances (such as not wanting to know a diagnosis of terminal illness), but usually people feel that they are entitled to information which affects their health. They may not always ask for it, for a number of reasons such as anxiety and worry, a feeling of being intimidated by a health professional or a clinical setting, or fearing to appear stupid by asking a silly question. However, when asked, people frequently express dissatisfaction with the amount of health information they have received, and this is particularly borne out by studies of patients in hospital and clinics.[13]

Health Education is the Basis for Health Promotion

Without education for health knowledge and understanding, there can be no informed decisions and actions to promote health. Decisions about the prevention of ill-health, recovery from illness and coping with chronic ill-health and disability should be made on the basis of a sound understanding and knowledge about health. Knowledge is power, and without health knowledge, people are powerless to change their health themselves because they do not have the knowledge of alternatives and therefore cannot make informed health choices. Thus health education is a tool which enables people to take more control over their own health, and over the factors which affect their health. This includes their physical and social environment (such as their place of work, or living conditions) as well as their personal habits and life-style. Health education is not only the process by which knowledge is obtained, but it is also the process by which values and attitudes are explored, decisions are made and action is taken. Health education can help people to become self-empowered, and thus to help themselves — and others — towards a healthier life.[14]

Health Education gets Results

It is obviously not true that health education has always achieved its goals — perhaps because the goals were unrealistic, the methods crude and under-developed and the health educators under-resourced. No professional practice can claim 100% success. But it is clear that in theory, a great deal of our major contemporary health problems are preventable, and that there is considerable scope for prevention and health promotion.[15] Health education is an essential and intrinsic part of prevention and health promotion.

It is also clear that health education in practice is successful in many cases of health promotion, primary prevention, and when it is part of the treatment and care of sick patients. This results in an improved quality of life and — more pragmatically — in savings for the health service.

Many examples could be quoted,[16] but the following success stories illustrate the point that health education is worth doing because it *works*. It gets results — for the consumer and for the health professional.

Health education success stories

Education to stop smoking

A study of 2,138 cigarette smokers attending the surgeries of 28 general practitioners in five group practices in London found that when GPs spent just a couple of minutes advising patients to stop smoking there were immediate changes in motivation and intention to stop smoking. Of the group who received advice, 3.3% were still not smoking a year later compared with 0.3% of a group who did not receive such advice. Although the success rate may appear low, the authors of this study point out that if all GPs in the UK participated in such an exercise, at the end of the year more than half a million people would have given up smoking.[17]

Prevention of unexpected infant deaths

A scheme started in Sheffield in 1972 has been largely responsible for a reduction in the rate of "possibly preventable deaths" in infants from 5.2 per 1,000 in 1972 to 1.9 per 1,000 in 1980. The scheme involved the identification of babies particularly at risk, and included frequent visits to these families by health visitors. There was also community health education work to prevent over-concentration on bottle-feeds, which was found to be a widespread problem. The implication of this study is that informal health education by health visitors is cost-effective, and effective in reducing infants deaths.[18]

Promotion of non-smoking

The activities of Bristol-based pressure groups GASP (Group Against Smoking in Public) and AGHAST (Action Group to Halt Advertising and Sponsorship by Tobacco) have led to an increase in no-smoking areas in restaurants, and to curtailment of tobacco sponsorship of sports and cultural events in the Bristol area.[19]

Changes in food labelling

Pressure on manufacturers has led to more information labels on consumer products such as foods and over-the-counter medicines. There is a trend to provide more information about the nutritional content of foods and to reduce medical "jargon" when describing medicines so that lay people will have a better understanding of their use.

Increasing knowledge about ante-natal care

In 1981 the West Midlands health services placed in local newspapers a series of full-page advertisements about keeping healthy during pregnancy. A follow-up study of over 100 women readers, and two control groups, showed that the advertisements had effected a significant change in understanding about self-care and the use of health services in pregnancy at an estimated cost of

continued on next page

continued

22p per woman. It was found that people liked the advertisements and found them helpful, and over 1,000 readers asked for further information by returning a coupon in the advertisement.[20]

A Personal Rationale for Health Education

We have expressed the basic reasons for health education in broad terms—but lofty philosophies need to be translated into everyday terms. So this section is to help each health professional to clarify her own personal reasons for undertaking health education in her daily work.

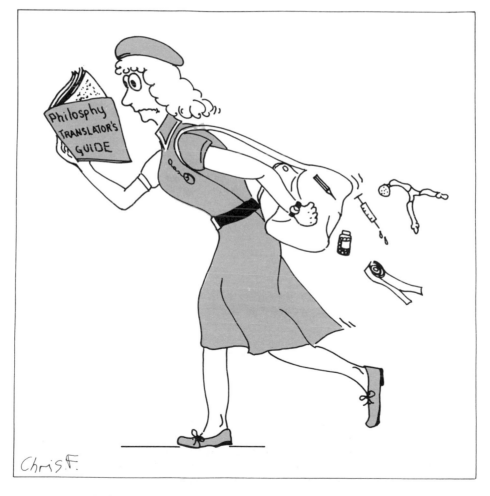

Lofty philosophies need to be translated into everyday terms!

Exercise — A personal rationale for health education

1. Spend a few minutes thinking about the specific health education tasks you undertake. Identify the range of tasks, clients/patients and health topics you cover.

2. Make a list of *all the reasons you can think of* for doing health education in your work.
   Reasons will vary according to profession and individual work, but they could include the following:
   — people have a right to know as much as I do about their health;
   — it helps people to get the most out of life;
   — it prevents unnecessary ill-health;
   — it increases people's ability to help themselves and be less dependent on me and my colleagues;
   — if people understand what's wrong with them they worry less;
   — people ask me questions and want to know;
   — patients recover more quickly if you explain their treatment to them so that they follow instructions properly;
   — it raises awareness of health hazards;
   — patients and relatives need help to understand medical advice;
   — so that people make the best use of the health services;
   — if I spend time health educating people, those people in turn will educate others;
   — to give people a sound basis for making health choices.

3. Try to summarize your personal rationale for health education by completing the following sentence:
   I believe that health education is an important part of my work because . . .
   (if you find this difficult, you might find it helpful to complete these two sentences first:
   I believe in health because . . .
   I believe in education because . . .)

The following case studies illustrate how two different health professionals may perceive the rationale for the health education aspects of their jobs.

Case studies — rationale for health education

Jean — A hospital nurse

Jean is a staff nurse on a women's surgical ward. Sheila is a patient who has been admitted for a hysterectomy; she is tense and anxious because she has never had an operation before, and all she can think of are scary stories about how awful she will feel. She is also worried about how quickly she will get

continued on next page

continued

back to normal afterwards, and whether she will be able to cope with her job in a supermarket and the care of her two children.

Jean believes it is her job and that of her colleagues to help Sheila to understand all about her operation and the effect it will have on her; she believes that Sheila has a right to this information and should be encouraged to think of herself as an active participant in her treatment and recovery. Jean also knows that knowledge helps to dispel fear, eases tension and consequently helps to lessen pain, and that teaching on self-care will help to make recovery as quick and easy as possible.

So Jean undertakes the following health education:
— ensuring that Sheila understands why she is having an operation;
— explaining what Sheila is likely to feel like when she ''comes round'', and how much pain or discomfort she is likely to experience;
— making sure that Sheila knows she can ask for pain-killers if she wants them;
— finding out from Sheila how much physical work she normally does and explaining to her how much it is advisable to do at first and how to increase the demands gradually until she returns to normal;
— teaching Sheila how to cope with the operation scar when she leaves hospital;
— explaining to Sheila about resuming her normal sexual relations after the operation;
— ensuring that Sheila feels free to ask about anything else she wants to know.

John — An occupational health doctor

John is a doctor in an occupational health service based in a large factory. He is concerned at the number of employees he sees with stress-related conditions such as high blood pressure, severe headaches, indigestion, ulcers, heavy drinking and anxiety states.

John believes that a great deal of this ill-health is preventable if conditions at work were improved and people could learn how to cope with stress, such as practising relaxation, taking more active physical recreation and learning to recognize, and change, their own responses to potentially stressful situations. His view is that they have a right to know how they can help themselves towards better health, and a right to discuss the health-damaging aspects of their working environment. He also feels that the management have an obligation to consider the health of the workforce in their policies and plans, and to ensure that the working environment is as health-promoting as possible, even if this means the occasional sacrifice of some profit.

So John's health education work includes:
— discussion with management and trade union officials to identify and minimize causes of stress at work;
— lunchtime group meetings for employees on ''coping with stress'' which include identifying stress symptoms, and working out coping strategies;
— after-work fitness and exercise groups;
— counselling sessions for individuals with particular problems.

Notes, References and Further Reading

1   For further reading on the concept of health see:

Wilson M (1976) *Health is for People*. London: Darton, Longman & Todd

Council for the Education and Training of Health Visitors (1977) *An Investigation into the Principles of Health Visiting*, pp 20-21

Stott N C H (1983) *Primary Health Care—Bridging the Gap between Theory and Practice*. Berlin/Heidelberg: Springer-Verlag, pp 33-43

2   This exercise is adapted with kind permission, from:

The Open University (1980) *The Good Health Guide*. Harmondsworth: Pan Books, p 16 (first published by Harper & Row)

3   British Market Research Bureau, for the Health Education Council, London (1977) *The "Cue" File on Positive Health*

4   The idea for this analysis is based on the findings of a French study on lay people's concept of health:

Herzlich C (1973) *Health and Illness*. European Monographs in Social Psychology. London: Academic Press

5   Hunt S M & McEwan J (1980) The development of a subjective health indicator. *Sociology of Health and Illness*, **2**(3)

6   This issue is dealt with extensively in medical sociology literature, for example:

Robinson D (1971) *The Process of Becoming Ill*. London: Routledge & Kegan Paul

Tuckett D (1976) *An Introduction to Medical Sociology*. London: Tavistock Publications, Ch 5

Zola I K (1978) Pathways to the Doctor. In Tuckett D Kaufert J M (eds) *Basic Readings in Medical Sociology*. London: Tavistock Publications, Ch 14

7   World Health Organisation Constitution 1948

8   Wilson M (1976) *Health is for People*. London: Darton, Longman & Todd, p 117

9   The "radiating circle" model is taken from:

Burkitt A (1982) Providing education about health. *Nursing*, June, 29-30

Reproduced by permission of Medical Education (International) Ltd

10   Townsend P & Davidson N (1982) *Inequalities in Health—The Black Report*. Harmondsworth: Pelican Books

Graham H (1984) *Women, Health and the Family*. Wheatsheaf Books

11   For analyses of the determinants of health, and the role of the health services in particular, see:

Cochrane A L (1972) *Effectiveness and Efficiency—Random Reflections on Health Services*. Nuffield Provincial Hospital Trust

Illich I (1977) *Limits to Medicine—Medical Nemesis: the Expropriation of Health*. Harmondsworth: Pelican Books

Horrobin D F (1978) *Medical Hubris.* Edinburgh: Churchill Livingstone
   (Horrobin's book is a reply to Illich's arguments in *Limits to Medicine.*)

Inglis B (1981) *Diseases of Civilisation.* London: Hodder & Stoughton

McKeown T (1979) *The Role of Medicine: Dream, Mirage or Nemesis.* Oxford:
   Blackwell

Thunhurst C (1982) *It Makes You Sick — The Politics of the NHS.* London: Pluto
   Press

Mitchell J (1984) *What is to be done about Illness and Health?* Harmondsworth:
   Penguin Books

For a teachers' manual, designed for use in schools, which looks at political, social
and individual determinants of health, see:

Dorn N & Nortoft B (1982) *Health Careers.* London: Institute for the Study of
   Drug Dependence

For a European view see:

O'Neill P (1983) *Health Crisis 2000.* London: Heinemann, for the World Health
   Organisation

12 World Health Organisation (1978) *Report on the Primary Health Care Conference,
   Alma Ata.*

This conference affirmed that health, and primary health care, is a fundamental
human right. It also affirmed that people have a right to be fully involved,
individually and collectively, in the planning and implementation of their health
care, and that primary health care includes health education.

13 See, for example:

Royal Commission on the National Health Service (1978) *Patients' Attitudes to the
   Hospital Service. Research Paper No 5.* London: HMSO

14 For an excellent review of the concept of education for self-empowerment, see:

Hopson B & Scally M (1981) *Lifeskills Teaching.* Maidenhead: McGraw-Hill, Ch 3

15 For more on the subject of prevention, see:

Department of Health and Social Security (1976). *Prevention and Health —
   Everybody's Business.* London: HMSO

Grey J M (1979) *Man Against Disease.* Oxford University Press

Royal College of General Practitioners, *Reports from General Practice:*
   No 18 (1981) *Health and Prevention in Primary Care*
   No 19 (1981) *Prevention of Arterial Disease in General Practice*
   No 20 (1981) *Prevention of Psychiatric Disorders in General Practice*

Royal College of General Practitioners, *Occasional Paper* No 22 (1983) *Promoting
   Prevention.*

Griffiths J, Dennis J, Draper P & Popay J (1983) Concepts of prevention. In
Clark J & Henderson J (eds) *Community Health.* Edinburgh: Churchill Livingstone,
   Ch 3

16 For many more summaries of evaluated studies of the effectiveness (or otherwise!)
of health education, see:

Bell J & Billington R (1980) *An Annoted Bibliography of Health Education Research, 1948-1978.* Edinburgh: Scottish Health Education Unit

Gatherer A Parfit J & Vessey M (1979) *Is Health Education Effective?* London: Health Education Council

Tones B K (1978) *Effectiveness and Efficiency in Health Education.* Edinburgh: Scottish Health Education Unit

Ewles L & Shipster P (1981) *One-to-One Health Education.* East Sussex Area Health Authority (now published by the South East Thames Regional Health Authority), pp 13-17

Wilson-Barnett J (1983) *Patient Teaching.* Edinburgh: Churchill Livingstone, pp 201-220

17   Russell M A H, Wilson C, Taylor C & Baker C D (1979) Effects of general practitioners' advice against smoking. *Br Med J*, 231-235

18   Carpenter R G *et al* (1983) Prevention of unexpected infant death. *Lancet*, 2 April, 723-727

19   Naidoo J (1983) GASP—a new anti-smoking initiative. *J Inst Hlth Educ*, **21**(1)

Report (1983) *AGHAST, GASP and the Right ANSR.* In Notes and News, *Lancet*, 30 July

20   Berry J M (1984) The impact of newspaper advertising on a regional antenatal campaign. *Hlth Educ J*, **43**(1)

Chapter 2
Principles
of Health
Education

Summary

The chapter begins with consideration of the meaning of education in terms of the health educator's range of methods and educational objectives, with examples and exercises. This is followed by an analysis of health education goals, and an exercise. The next section, on the concept of health education, highlights some of the important issues to be considered. Primary, secondary and tertiary health education are described, and the final section summarises 7 dimensions of health education, and discusses the difficulties of defining health education and health promotion.

The previous chapter focused on *health*; we now move on to consider the meaning of *education* and *health education*.

The Meaning of "Education"

Volumes have been written on the philosophy and concept of education, but our specific concern here is to explore what "education" means in the context of the health professional's work as a health educator.

Exercise — What does "education" mean to you?

Answer *yes* or *no* to the following.
A health professional is engaged in health education when she is:
1. Instructing a patient when to take his tablets   _____
2. Advising a mother about feeding her toddler   _____
3. Answering questions about childbirth from a group of
    pregnant women   _____
4. Showing a diabetic how to give himself an injection   _____
5. Persuading a determined smoker to stop smoking   _____

continued on next page

continued

6. Leading a discussion on sexual relationships with a group of 16-year-olds   _____

7. Describing the pros and cons of vaccination to a baby's parents   _____

8. Helping a woman to decide whether to have an abortion   _____

9. Listening to a recently bereaved widower talking about his late wife   _____

10. Asking a group of new mothers how they feel about motherhood   _____

11. Warning a heavy drinker about the dangers of alcohol   _____

12. Explaining the case for more play facilities to her local councillor   _____

13. Teaching a routine of physical exercises to a keep-fit class   _____

If you answered *no* to any of these questions, try to identify why you think that particular activity is not "education".

A number of different activities have been identified in this exercise, including instructing, advising, explaining, listening, leading discussion, and helping a client to make a decision. This illustrates that the term "education", in the context of a health educator's work, has a far broader meaning than the traditional concept of formal classroom teaching.

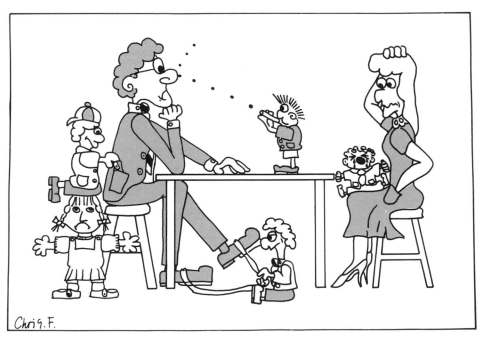

A health professional is engaged in health education when she is explaining the case for more play facilities to her local councillor!

Not only is there a range of different activities within health education, but also a range of different objectives. This is explored below.

Types of Educational Objectives

In the exercise *What does education mean to you?*, Q.3 "Answering questions about childbirth" has the objective that the mothers know about childbirth; Q.6 "Leading a discussion on sexual relationships" has the objective of helping the teenagers to work out their ideas and attitudes in this area; Q.4 "Showing a diabetic how to give himself an injection" has the objective that he acquires the skill of injecting himself. This illustrates that there are three kinds of objectives: what the educator would like the clients to *know*, *feel* and *do* as a result of the education (these can also be referred to as cognitive, affective and behavioural objectives).[1]

Objectives about "Knowing"

These objectives are concerned with giving information, explaining it, ensuring that the client understands it, and thus increasing the client's knowledge.

In the exercise, instructing the patient when to take his tablets has the objective that the patient will *know* when to take his tablets. Similarly, explaining the pros and cons of vaccination has the objective that the baby's parents will then *know* what the advantages and disadvantages of vaccination are.

Objectives about "Feeling"

These objectives are concerned with attitudes, beliefs, values and opinions. All these are complex concepts, studied extensively by psychologists.[2] However, the important feature to note now is that they are all concerned with people's *feelings*, often with strong feelings. For example, attitudes are a combination of concepts, information and emotion. If a person has a particular attitude it means that he is likely to respond in a particular way. So someone with the attitude that cleanliness is next to godliness is likely to respond to a neighbour's dirty house with distaste or even disgust.

Objectives about "feelings" are concerned with clarifying, forming or changing the clients attitudes, beliefs, values or opinions.

In the exercise, listening to the recently-bereaved widower has the objective that the client *feels* less distressed by enabling him to express his feelings of grief. Asking a group of new mothers how they feel about motherhood has the objective that they *feel* less isolated and less tense through sharing their feelings, learning that there are others in the same situation who feel the same way, and getting practical help and emotional support from each other.

Objectives about "Doing"

These objectives are concerned with the client's skills and actions. In the exercise, teaching a routine of physical exercises had the objective that people acquire the skills and use them.

In health education, educational objectives are rarely concerned exclusively with knowing, feeling or doing—a mixture is usually required. For example, in the exercise, when advising a mother about feeding her toddler, the health educator probably has several objectives in mind:

—the objective of ensuring that the mother *knows* which foods are nourishing for her child and which are best given in restricted amounts;
—the objective of changing the mother's erroneous *belief* that sugar is essential to give her child energy, and *relieving her anxiety* that her healthy child's "food fads" may cause serious ill-health;
—the objective that the mother learns what to *do* at mealtimes when her child has a tantrum over eating his food.

Thus the health educator is concerned with what the mother *knows*, *feels*, and *does* about feeding her toddler.

There is a mixture of objectives implicit in some of the other examples too. Persuading a determined smoker to stop smoking is primarily concerned with the objective of changing the smoker's feeling of determination to continue into a feeling of wanting to stop. This could lead to the "doing" objective of acquiring the skills necessary to stop smoking (such as being able to refuse the offer of a cigarette). "Knowing" objectives may be involved, too, concerned with giving the smoker information about the effects of smoking and various approaches to stopping smoking.

Exercise — Identifying types of educational objectives

Identify the *knowing*, *feeling* and *doing* objectives which the health educator may have in these situations:
1. Helping a woman to decide whether to have an abortion.
2. Warning a heavy drinker about the dangers of alcohol.
3. Explaining the case for more play facilities to a local councillor.

It is apparent that the range of objectives which the health educator may be trying to achieve is very wide, and it is helpful to consider all these objectives in broad categories, which we have called *health education goals*.

Health Education Goals

Health Consciousness Goal

The goal here is to raise health consciousness, or awareness, of health issues. Some "knowing" objectives will fall into this category, because they are concerned that people know (however vaguely) something about a health issue.

Knowledge Goal

Obviously, the objectives in this category are all "knowing" ones, because the goal is to give specific knowledge and information about the health issues which people are already aware of, but about which they have little real knowledge or understanding.

Self-awareness Goal

The objectives in this category are "feeling" ones, concerned with exploring feelings and being aware of one's feelings in relation to a particular health issue or to health in general. It may involve clarifying values about health—in other words, helping people to identify what is really important to them.

Attitude Change Goal

Objectives in this category are "feeling" ones, concerned with changing what people feel, what they believe and what their opinion is.

Decision-making Goal

This involves both "knowing" and "feeling" objectives, and is concerned with deciding what to do in the future about health or a particular aspect of health. The decision is based on knowledge of relevant information and understanding of the feelings and values involved.

Behaviour Change Goal

"Doing" objectives fall into this category, because the goal is concerned with carrying out a decision and actually doing something about a health matter.

Social Change Goal

This is the rather complex goal of making "healthy choices easier choices" by changing the physical and/or social environment so that people are encouraged to adopt healthier behaviour. Ultimately, decisions about changing the environment are made and carried out by people who make policies and plans, such as health authority members and officers, local councillors and MPs. It may be necessary to work through a number of "knowing", "feeling" and "doing" objectives with these people in order to achieve the goal of social change. It may also be necessary to work through them with members of the public in order to gain support for the proposed change.

The examples overleaf illustrate these goals in relation to education about alcohol and exercise.

There are important points to consider about these goals. The first is that the order in which the goals are listed should not be taken to imply that people necessarily progress through them in turn. For example, people may change their attitude towards exercise *after* they have experienced the benefits—they may not initially think that exercise is a good thing (ie. they may have a negative attitude towards it) but if they are reluctantly coerced into taking some, and then discover that they feel better as a result and actually enjoy it, then the attitude change will *follow*. So in this case the behaviour change came before the attitude change.[2]

Health education goals — Examples

Goal	Alcohol education	Exercise education
Health consciousness	I know that drinking too much is bad for me.	I know that exercise is supposed to be healthy.
Knowledge	I know the effects of alcohol on me.	I know that exercise aids physical stamina, suppleness and strength, and makes the heart stronger.
Self-awareness	I'm aware that I'm drinking too much and I'm a bit worried about it.	I feel unfit because I get out of breath easily and I'd like to feel fitter.
Attitude change	I now believe it's important to change my drinking habits.	I used to believe that exercise was only for health freaks but now I believe I would feel better if I did more exercise.
Decision-making	I will limit my drinking to three pints a day.	I'll join a keep-fit class.
Behaviour change	I now drink less than I used to.	I go to a keep-fit class and I'm generally more physically active — I walk rather than take a bus sometimes, climb stairs and avoid lifts, and take my neighbour's dog for walks.
Social change	Higher taxation on alcohol. Soft drinks more socially acceptable in pubs. Stricter controls on under-age drinking. Alcohol less easy to buy (e.g. at supermarkets). Alcohol advertising banned.	Sports facilities cheaper and more available. Showers at work so people can run/cycle to work or in lunch hours. School gyms and swimming pools open for adults in evenings and at weekends. Lunchtime and after-work group classes/runs.

The second point is that achieving one goal does not necessarily mean that there will be progress to another. For example, most smokers know that "smoking is bad for you" and actually wish they didn't smoke—but this has not led on to a real decision *not* to smoke, nor to the change in behaviour from smoking to not smoking. People's attitudes are frequently incompatible with their behaviour.

Thirdly, it is important to be aware that different goals are appropriate for different people, and the health educator needs to take this into account. For example, people who come to a Weight-watchers group have already made the decision to try to do something about their weight problem; they do not need their consciousness raised about it. But in other situations there may be a need to raise awareness of a health issue; for example, new mothers may be totally unaware that leaving babies alone to feed themselves with a bottle is dangerous because the baby could choke.

Finally, there are different health education strategies appropriate for these different goals, and these are considered in detail in Chapter 7.

Exercise — Identifying health education goals

Look back at the *Examples of Health Education Goals*.
Choose a different health education topic, for example, family planning, food hygiene, home safety education, or coping with children's tantrums.
Identify the goals you might have for education about your topic.

Exploring the Concept of Health Education

We have now seen that both health and education are broad concepts, open to a variety of interpretations by different people, so it is not surprising that there is no satisfactory definition of "health education".[3] However, it is important for each health professional to explore the dimensions, scope and boundaries of health education, and to arrive at her own view of what "health education" means for her in the context of her own professional practice.

The exercise on the next page is designed to help the reader to explore the concept of health education.[4]

The statements in this exercise raise important issues, which are discussed briefly here, and explored in greater depth in other chapters.

Agreement with Statements 2 and 3 implies that health education is not just about physical health, but about mental and emotional health as well. Agreement with Statement 4 means facing the difficulty that not all health professionals are perfect pictures of radiant health, and may have unhealthy habits of one sort or another.

Statements 8 and 11 raise the controversial question of whether health educators know what is best for people and should try to get them to adopt the sort of life-style which professionals consider "healthy", or whether the health professional's aim is to encourage people to make up their own minds, even if this means going against medical advice.

Exercise — Exploring the concept of health education

Consider each of the following statements, and decide whether you agree or disagree with each statement:

		Agree	Disagree
1.	Health education is a life-long process from birth to death	‾‾‾	‾‾‾
2.	Health education includes giving people information about the way their bodies work	‾‾‾	‾‾‾
3.	Health education includes helping people to recognize and express their emotions appropriately	‾‾‾	‾‾‾
4.	Health education should be taught by the example of health educators, as well as their words	‾‾‾	‾‾‾
5.	Health education includes helping healthy people to learn about preventing health problems	‾‾‾	‾‾‾
6.	Health education includes instructing people how to carry out their doctor's orders	‾‾‾	‾‾‾
7.	Health education includes making people aware that social and financial conditions affect health and life expectancy	‾‾‾	‾‾‾
8.	Health education aims to change people's behaviour and lifestyles, such as taking more exercise and not smoking	‾‾‾	‾‾‾
9.	Health education includes getting people together to fight for changes in health policy	‾‾‾	‾‾‾
10.	Health education includes helping families to learn how to cope with a sick member	‾‾‾	‾‾‾
11.	Health education includes enabling people to reach their own decisions in health matters	‾‾‾	‾‾‾
12.	Health education includes making people aware that advertising and the mass media shape their options in health matters	‾‾‾	‾‾‾

Statements 7, 9 and 12 draw attention away from the individual consumer of health education to the society in which that consumer lives. This raises another controversial issue in health education—whether educating people about health includes looking at root causes of ill-health, such as poverty, and working to change conditions which are associated with ill-health rather than changing the individual to survive the conditions.

Statements 5, 6 and 10 are about identifying the consumers of health education, and whether health education is confined to prevention for the healthy, or whether it is useful for patients whose illness or disability has not been prevented. Related to this is the idea of primary, secondary and tertiary health education.

Primary, Secondary and Tertiary Health Education

The framework of primary, secondary and tertiary health education is a useful one, based on the concept of primary, secondary and tertiary prevention in community medicine.[5]

Examples — Primary, secondary and tertiary health education

	Nutrition	Road Accidents
Primary health education	Education about adequate and balanced food providing enough nutrients, fibre and energy.	Accident prevention, including campaigning for safer roads and vehicles, as well as educating individuals about safe practices.
Secondary health education	How to adjust habits in cases of overweight or other reversible health problems, such as maturity-onset diabetes.	How to give first aid after an accident to maximize chances of full recovery.
Tertiary health education	How to adjust eating habits to ensure maximum health and minimum complications in chronic incurable conditions, such as juvenile-onset diabetes or food allergies.	Rehabilitation training to maximize potential for healthy living following accident causing permanent disability, such as loss of a limb or paralysis.

Primary health education is directed at healthy people, and aims to prevent ill-health arising in the first place. Most health education for children and young people falls into this category, dealing with such topics as hygiene, contraception, nutrition and personal relationships. Primary health education is concerned not merely with helping to prevent illness, but with positively improving the quality of health and thus the quality of life.

There is also often a major role for health education when a person is ill. It may be possible to prevent ill-health moving to a chronic or irreversible stage, and to restore the person to his former state of health. This is known as *secondary* health education—educating patients about their condition and what to do about it. Restoring good health may involve the patient in changing his behaviour (such as stopping smoking) or in complying with a therapeutic regime and, possibly, learning about self-care and self-help. Clearly, health education of the patient is of great importance if his treatment and therapy are to be effective and if his illness is not to recur.

But there are, of course, many patients whose ill-health has not been, or could not be, prevented and who cannot be completely cured. There are also people with permanent disabilities and handicaps. *Tertiary* health education for such clients is concerned with educating the patient and his relatives about how to make the most of the remaining potential for healthy living, and how to avoid unnecessary hardships, restrictions and complications. Rehabilitation programmes contain a considerable amount of tertiary health education.

However, it is not always easy to see where people fit into this primary, secondary or tertiary framework, because, as we have already seen, a person's state of health is open to interpretation. For example, is educating an overweight person who feels perfectly well despite the overweight *primary* or *secondary* health education?

We have now identified and discussed a number of dimensions of health education, which are summarized in the following section.

Seven Dimensions of Health Education

1. Health, and therefore health education, is concerned with the whole person, and encompasses physical, mental, social, emotional, spiritual and societal aspects.
2. Health education is a life-long process from birth to death, helping people to change and adapt at all stages (from sperm to worm!).
3. Health education is concerned with people at all points of health and illness, from the completely healthy to the chronically sick and handicapped, to maximize each person's potential for healthy living.
4. Health education is directed towards individuals, families, groups and whole communities.
5. Health education is concerned with helping people to help themselves and with helping people to work towards creating healthier conditions for everybody, "making healthy choices easier choices".
6. Health education involves formal and informal teaching and learning using a range of methods.
7. Health education is concerned with a range of goals, including giving information, attitude change, behaviour change and social change.

This broad view of health education means that there are many grey areas of work where it is difficult to say whether the work should or should not be labelled health education. For example, is teaching a patient about a therapeutic diet "treatment" or "education"? Is behaviour modification "therapy" or "education"? A more important question, though, is whether the label matters—and we believe it doesn't.

However, it should be recognized that health education is often taken to mean a much narrower field of activity. Sometimes it is taken to mean primary prevention only, and concern with patient education, for example, is excluded. Sometimes it only refers to formal teaching with individuals and groups, excluding all the learning which goes on from, for example, television, friends and family. Finally, health education is frequently interpreted in the sense that it only refers to education which aims to change people's behaviour. This excludes work for other goals, such as changing the environment into a healthier place.

Another cause of current confusion is the use of the term "health promotion". This has been used more frequently in the last few years, and indeed some Health Authorities now employ Health Promotion Officers. Often, "health promotion" is used as an umbrella term which includes traditional health education, but sometimes it is used in more specific ways. It may refer to the marketing/advertising aspects of health education, or to the political aspects of lobbying for changes in health policy or legislation, or to changing health policies at local level. Finally, it is sometimes used to refer to the emphasis on positive health, as opposed to the negatively-flavoured prevention of ill-health.

We are more concerned with exploring the territory of health education than with drawing rigid boundaries and we hope that the lack of rigid boundaries will aid the integration of health education into the everyday work of all health professionals.

Notes, References and Further Reading

1 For further reading on educational aims and objectives, see:

Kelly A V (1977) *The Curriculum: Theory and Practice.* London: Harper & Row, Ch 6

Two classic works on educational objectives are:

Bloom B S *et al* (1956) *Taxonomy of Educational Objectives.* London: Longmans

Mager R (1962) *Preparing Instructional Objectives.* Fearon

For a critical discussion on the use of educational objectives, see:

Stenhouse L (1975) *An Introduction to Curriculum Research and Development.*
    London: Heinemann, Ch 6

2 An introductory book on the psychology of values, attitudes and behaviour change, and the relationship between the three, is:

Reich B & Adcock C (1976) *Values, Attitudes and Behaviour Change.* London:
    Methuen (Essential Psychology Series)

3 A list of definitions of health education can be found in:

Strehlow M S (1983) *Education for Health.* London: Harper & Row, pp 173-175

4 Based on an exercise "Health Education Is . . ." in the training manual for the Schools Health Education Project 5-13, published by the Health Education Council, London, and reproduced by kind permission of the Council.

5 For more on the subject of prevention, see the publications listed in item 15 of the Notes, References and Further Reading at the end of Chapter 1.

Chapter 3
Five Approaches to Health Education

Summary

Five approaches to health education are identified: medical, behaviour change, educational, client-directed and social change approaches. The key features of each are discussed, with examples of their application. Discussion about the use of different approaches in practice is followed by an exercise on analysing the philosophy of health education.

We have now seen that health education is a process which cannot be tied down and confined within a neat package. This has the danger of leaving health professionals in a state of confusion, unsure of what they are supposed to be doing in health education. It's easy to float off with our heads in the clouds, but we need to get back to earth and know where we are going. In order to help health professionals to decide on their own position, we identify five approaches to health education.[1]

The Medical and Behaviour Change Approaches

The Medical Approach

The aim of this approach is freedom from medically-defined disease and disability, such as infectious diseases, cancer and heart disease. The approach involves promoting medical intervention to prevent or ameliorate ill-health, generally using a persuasive and authoritarian method—for example, persuading parents to bring their children for immunization and vaccination, women to use family planning clinics and middle-aged men to be screened for high blood pressure.

The Behaviour Change Approach

The aim of this approach is to change people's attitudes and behaviour, so that they adopt a "healthy" life-style, and examples of it include the promotion of the attitude that smoking is antisocial, teaching people how to stop smoking, education about "sensible" drinking, encouraging people to take more exercise, look after their teeth,

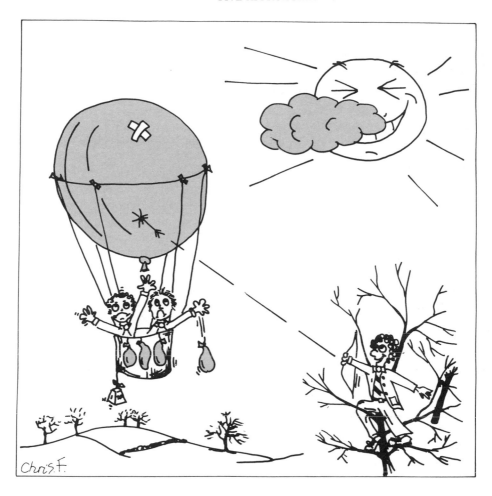

It's easy to float off with our heads in the clouds, but we need to get back down to earth
and know where we are going!

eat the "right" foods and so on. The *medical* and *behavioural change* approaches are
often loosely referred to as "prevention" or "the medical model", and they often
overlap (eg. using medical facilities like a screening service or a family planning clinic
is a behaviour change).

Proponents of these approaches argue that medical and health experts have the
knowledge which enables them to know what is in the best interests of their patients
and the public at large, and that it is their responsibility to persuade people to adopt
the "healthiest" measures. Furthermore, society has vested that responsibility with
them, and people often seek advice and help in health matters. It is not necessarily
a matter of persuading clients against their will; indeed, people often ask to be
persuaded, even bullied, into doing things they find difficult, such as stopping smoking
or losing weight. A further point in favour of these approaches is that the individuals
concerned may not be in a position to take responsibility for themselves, for example,
because they are too young, too ill, or are mentally handicapped.

These approaches have been embodied in much traditional health education of the prescriptive kind. Recently, though, they have been the subject of much criticism, on the following grounds.

— They assume that lay people believe that the "experts" know best. This is a dubious assumption, particularly in the light of controversial issues when the experts have been seen to change their minds or give conflicting advice, as in the disputes over whether butter or unsaturated fat is better for you, whether jogging does more harm than good, and in revising the message that carrots and apples are good for cleaning your teeth.
— They involve the imposition of medical values on the client. Frequently, this means the imposition of middle-class values on working-class people, and the ethical justification for this is doubtful. For example, losing weight and lowering blood pressure may be the most important thing to a doctor, but drinking beer in the pub with friends may be far more important to his overweight, middle-aged, unemployed patient. Who is to say which set of values is "right"—the doctor or his patient? Whose life is it anyway?
— They may induce feelings of guilt if the client chooses not to follow the prescribed "healthy" regime.
— They may induce rebelliousness in people who are fed up with being told what to do.
— They assume that individual behaviour is the primary cause of ill-health. This is a limited view—as we have seen when looking at the determinants of health—and it is argued that focusing on the individual distracts attention from the more important (and politically sensitive) determinants of health such as socio-economic conditions and unemployment.
— They also assume that individuals have a genuine freedom to choose "healthy" life-styles, but the truth is that freedom to choose is often limited. Economic factors may affect the choice of food because, for example, fresh fruit and wholemeal bread are relatively more expensive than biscuits and white bread. Social factors are also important: there is very little real freedom of choice about smoking for an adolescent whose parents and friends all smoke, and who risks ridicule if he does not; and smoking may be one of the few routes of escape to relaxation in an overcrowded house in an inner-city area. Also, how much freedom do people really have to change other health-demoting factors such as stressful working conditions and unemployment? This approach to health education has been called "victim-blaming" because it blames people for their own ill-health when in fact they are the victims of their circumstances. In situations where resources of time, energy and income are limited, health choices become health compromises. What a health professional may see as irresponsibility is actually what the client sees as the most responsible action in the circumstances.[2]

The Educational Approach

The aim of this approach is to give knowledge and ensure understanding of health issues, based on the notion that this will enable well-informed decisions to be made and acted upon. Information about health is presented in as value-free a way as possible, and people are helped to explore their values and attitudes, and to make their own decisions about their health behaviour. Help in carrying out those decisions may also be offered.

The essential differences between this approach and the previous ones is that it does not seek to impose the educator's own ideas or to persuade people; the educator must be able to accept that clients' decisions may well not be those that the educator would have preferred.

Examples of this approach are recent schemes of health education in schools, such as the Schools Health Education Project for 5 to 18-year-olds,[3] and the Open University's Health Choices course.[4]

This approach, too, has its strengths and limitations. It may attempt to be value-free, but no educational process can claim to be totally value-free. The initial choice of health education materials and methods is, in itself, based on the value judgement of the health educator. Furthermore, the health educator obviously has her own views, which are likely to become apparent in many subtle (and perhaps not-so-subtle) ways.

However, this approach is less open to the criticisms of imposing medical/middle class values, and making the assumption that the "expert" has the "right" answers, since, in this approach, people are required to decide for themselves what the "right" answers are. It can still be criticized on the grounds that it focuses on the individual, and takes little account of changing the socio-economic environment which restricts the individual's freedom of choice.

The Client-directed Approach

The focus of this approach is on working with clients in order that they can identify what they want to know about, and make their own decisions and choices according to their own interests and values. The essential difference between the client-directed approach and the others discussed above is that concerns are identified by the *clients*, not by the educator.

Examples of the client-directed approach to health education can be found in the work of the women's movement. Groups of women decide collectively what their health concerns are, and set up self-help groups to look at health issues such as the menopause or contraception. The emphasis is on identifying their *own* concerns, in contrast to the concerns identified by the medical profession, which is frequently also dominated by men and male values.[5]

The client-directed approach is also at the core of many community-based initiatives in health education, which aim to help people in communities to identify their health concerns and work towards their own solutions. A professional worker may act as a facilitator to help people to work together in the early stages. Such a worker may be a community social worker or a health professional with a specific brief to develop community projects.[6]

This approach also has its limitations. One problem is that clients may need to learn to be self-directing; their previous experience may have led them to expect and want professional leadership, and the lack of it may cause frustration, apathy and, ultimately, failure to get a project off the ground.

Secondly, there may be conflict between the identified concerns of the clients, and those of the professionals. For instance, a community may decide that its greatest health need is more high-technology medicine at the local hospital, whereas the health professionals may see a greater need for more basic primary health care facilities such as a domiciliary chiropody service for the elderly and more community nurses. However, a strength of this approach is that neither medical nor professional values are imposed upon clients.

The Social Change Approach

The aim of the social change approach is to change the environment to facilitate the choice of healthier life-styles—in other words, it aims to make healthy choices easier choices.

Using this approach involves political or social action. This action may be concerned with large issues of great political significance, such as the link between unemployment and ill-health, and supporting political action to lower the rate of unemployment. Or it may be concerned with issues on a much smaller and less politically-sensitive scale, such as the provision of wholemeal bread in schools and hospitals. In both these examples, the aim is to make the healthier option (having a job or eating wholemeal bread) an easier choice (by having more jobs available and having wholemeal bread on the menu). An important difference between the social change approach and the previous ones is that the health education is directed at policy-makers and planners at all levels, as well as at the general public.

The contentious nature of the social change approach is its chief limitation. Many of the issues are politically sensitive (eg. unemployment) and the health educator is likely to fall foul of powerful vested interest groups and financial considerations—for example, improving safety at work may involve introducing safety measures which reduce productivity and profit. The approach is also contentious because it is markedly different from traditional individual health education directed at clients. Its aim of effecting social change is difficult for some people to justify as "education", but we believe that raising awareness of the health aspects of policy decisions can be considered as valid education of policy-makers and the public.

These five approaches are summarized below, and illustrated with smoking as an example of how the different approaches could be used in anti-smoking health education.

Using Different Approaches in Practice

In our view, there is no one "right" approach to health education. We believe that each health professional should work out for herself which approach she uses in each situation, which one she feels accords most comfortably with her own professional code of conduct and which one is the most appropriate for her clients' needs. On the issue of smoking, for example, she may feel a strong moral obligation to use a persuasive behaviour-change approach with her clients; on the other hand, she may feel that she should use a client-directed approach and leave the topic alone unless the client wishes to discuss it. Or she may feel that the best use of her energies is lobbying locally for more no-smoking areas in public places.

A further important point is that each approach does not have to be considered in isolation from the others; it may well be appropriate to use a mix of approaches to tackle a particular issue. A health professional may decide to use a behaviour-change approach with a pregnant woman smoker who coughs and is therefore clearly putting her own and her child's health at risk; she may use an educational approach with a class of 12-year-olds who are not yet hooked on smoking, a client-directed approach with a women's health group, and a social-change approach when working to achieve a no-smoking policy in local health premises.

In summary, then, the reasons for identifying the five approaches we have discussed are:

—to enable health professionals to identify the range of different approaches to the current practice of health education;
—to enable the strengths and limitations of the different approaches to be understood;
—to help each health professional to identify her own approach in each situation, and to consider whether other approaches, or a mix of approaches, might be more appropriate or effective.

Five approaches to health education: Summary and example

	Aim	Health education activity	Example — anti-smoking
MEDICAL	Freedom from medically defined disease and disability.	Promotion of medical intervention to prevent or ameliorate ill-health.	Aim — freedom from lung disease, heart disease and other smoking-related disorders. Activity — encourage people to seek early detection and treatment of smoking related disorders.
BEHAVIOUR CHANGE	Individual behaviour conducive to freedom from disease.	Attitude and behaviour change to encourage adoption of ''healthier'' life-style.	Aim — behaviour changes from smoking to not smoking. Activity — persuasive education to prevent non-smokers starting and persuade smokers to stop.

continued on next page

continued

	Aim	Health education activity	Example — anti-smoking
EDUCATIONAL	Individuals with knowledge and understanding enabling well informed decisions to be made and acted upon.	Information about cause and effects of health-demoting factors. Exploration of values and attitudes. Development of skills required for healthy living.	Aim — clients will have understanding of the effects of smoking on health. They will make a decision about whether to smoke or not, and act on this decision. Activity — giving information to clients about the effects of smoking. Helping them to explore their own values and attitudes and come to a decision. Helping them to learn how to stop smoking if they want to.
CLIENT-DIRECTED	Working with clients on the clients' own terms.	Working with clients' identified health issues choices and actions.	Anti-smoking issue only considered if clients identify it as a concern. Clients identify what they want to know and do about it.
SOCIAL CHANGE	Physical and social environment enabling choice of healthier lifestyle	Political/ social action to change physical/ social environment.	Aim — make smoking socially un-acceptable, so it is easier not to smoke than to smoke. Activity — no-smoking policy in all public places. Cigarette sales less accessible, especially to children, and in hospital. Promotion of not smoking as social norm. Limiting and challenging smoking advertising and sports sponsorship.

Exercise — Analysing your philosophy of health education[7]

Consider the following statements A and B.

A. The aim of health education is to inform people about the ways in which their behaviour and lifestyle can affect their health, to ensure that the information is understood, to help them explore their values and attitudes, and (where appropriate) to help them to change their behaviour.

B. The aim of health education is to raise awareness of the many socio-economic policies at national and local level (eg. employment, housing, food subsidies, advertising, transport and health service policies) which are not conducive to good health, and to actively work towards a change in those policies.

1.   Taking Statement A:
     — list arguments in support of this view;
     — list any points about the limitations of this view, and any arguments against it.
2.   Do the same with Statement B.
3.   Do you think that the views in A and B are *complementary* or *incompatible?*
     Why?
4.   Imagine these two views at either end of a spectrum:

A | . . . . . | . . . . . | . . . . . | . . . . . | . . . . . | B
     1   2   3   4   5

Indicate the two positions on the scale of 1 to 5 which most closely reflect (a) *what you actually do* in practice and (b) *what you would like to do* if you were free to work exactly as you would wish to.

Notes, References and Further Reading

1   Many articles have been published in recent years on different approaches to, or models of, health education. Most of them have been critical of traditional health education aimed at changing the behaviour of individuals. Some notable articles and readings are:

Beattie A (1984) Health education and the science teacher: invitation to a debate. *Education and Health*, **2** (1)

Burkitt A (1983) Health education. In Clark J & Henderson J (eds) *Community Health*. Edinburgh: Churchill Livingstone, Ch 4

Draper P (1983) Tackling the disease of ignorance. *Self Health,* (1)

Mitchell J (1982) Looking after ourselves: an individual responsibility? *Roy Soc Hlth J,* (4)

Tones B K (1981) Health education: prevention or subversion? *Roy Soc Hlth J,* (3)

2 Graham H (1984) *Women, Health and the Family.* Wheatsheaf Books, Ch 12

3 Schools Health Education Project, funded jointly by the Schools Council and the Health Education Council. Material for 5–13-year-olds published by Nelson (1977) and for 13–18-year-olds published by Forbes (1982).

4 See, for example, the book which is part of the course materials:

The Open University (1980) *The Good Health Guide.* Harmonsworth: Pan Books (first published by Harper & Row)

5 A book on women's health which reflects this approach is: Phillips A & Rakusen J (1979) *Our Bodies Ourselves.* Harmondsworth: Penguin Books

6 The community development approach to health education is outlined in:

Hubley J (1980) Community development and health education. *J Inst Hlth Educ,* **18** (4)

7 This exercise is based on an idea in the training manual for the Schools Health Education Project 5–13, published by the Health Education Council, London, and is here reproduced by kind permission of the Council.

Chapter 4
Ethical Aspects of Health Education

Summary

Five major areas of ethical concern to the health educator are identified and discussed: the example set by the health educator, the balance of control and power between professional and client, individual responsibility versus social change, justification for intervention and conflicting interests. Some suggested guidelines on making ethical decisions are followed by two case studies where the reader is invited to consider the ethical questions raised.

Any professional activity which tries to affect the lives of other people poses ethical questions for the professional. What rights (if any) does she have to try to influence clients? Does trying to persuade people into healthier lifestyles merely serve to induce guilt and stress? What health messages should be published when expert opinion is likely to change? These, and other, questions pose real dilemmas for the health educator, and we have identified five major areas of ethical concern.

The Example of the Health Educator

Consider the cases of an overweight dietitian, a nurse who smokes and a GP who never takes exercise. All three are in a position where they will need to discuss these issues with patients, and possibly be asked for advice which they clearly do not follow themselves. Should they avoid the subject (which is probably impossible), try to hide their own problem (also probably impossible), pretend that they do not have a problem and maintian a professional distance, laugh it off, discuss their own problem with the patient, pretend they are actively trying to do something about their problem, or really try to solve the problem and become a shining example of healthiness? Most of these options are likely to increase the stress level of the educator and lower her credibility even further in the eyes of the client.

Few health educators would claim that they are perfect examples of healthy living, but we suggest that they have a professional responsibility to consider their own health and ways in which it could be improved. This is because:

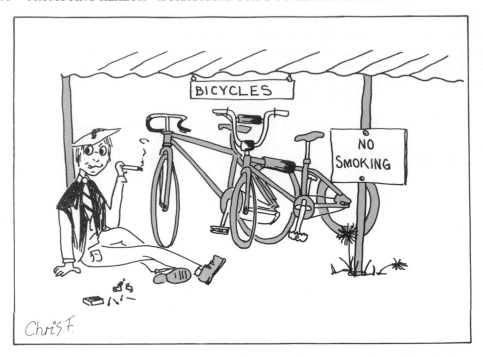

Few health educators would claim that they are perfect examples of healthy living!

—clients are more likely to accept help and advice from health professionals who set a good example;
—health professionals are teaching by example, and the examples cited above convey silent messages that it is OK to be overweight/smoke/take no exercise!

If there is an obvious health problem such as overweight, it is probably best to make an open and honest acknowledgement of it to the client, and use the experience to develop a more personal understanding of the client's difficulties.

Who is in Charge: Professional or Client?

A central issue for a health educator to consider is her underlying philosophy of education. It is useful to consider this as a spectrum of positions. At one end, there is coercion or persuasion of clients (eg. to stop smoking, take the prescribed tablets or seek the help of a marriage guidance counsellor). A slightly less forceful position is that of giving advice, and less forceful still is the neutral position of "giving the facts" but leaving the client to decide without trying to push him in either direction. At the least forceful end of the spectrum is the health professional who listens, gives information when asked but never offers advice or even an opinion. In essence, this is an issue of control and power—is it the professional or the client who is choosing the topic, directing the discussion and deciding about future behaviour? It may be argued that trying to persuade does no harm because people won't do what they don't want to do, but that may not be true for children or people who are not assertive about their own views.

Each health educator needs to decide for herself what is ethically acceptable in each situation. There is no "right" answer. It is arguable that persuasion is an unethical imposition of the professional's values on her clients, but it is equally arguable that not trying to persuade a client towards a healthier way of life is avoiding the professional responsibility of trying to improve people's health.

Individual Responsibility versus Social Change

As we discussed in Chapter 3, a great deal of traditional health education has aimed to change the behaviour of individuals towards healthier lifestyles. In other words, it aims to change people to fit the environment, and has done little to make the environment a healthier place to live in. It has also resulted in "blaming the victim" for his ill-health, which is an ethical issue the health educator needs to face. On the other hand, it can be argued that individuals often *can* do something to improve their own health, that they want to take responsibility for themselves and that health education is an essential tool in that process.

However, if a health professional chooses to use a social change approach, she faces a further dilemma when educational pressure becomes political action in the form of, for example, protest marches, demonstrations and active lobbying. Our view is that such political action is outside the scope of health education, although health educators are obviously free to participate in a private capacity. Some activities fall between the two poles of education and political action, and in these cases each health educator must make a decision in the light of her own philosophy. For example, should a health educator agree to publicise a meeting of a group of activists planning to demonstrate about the closure of a hospital?

Justification for Intervention

A common complaint from the public is that experts keep changing their minds, and there are many examples which illustrate the truth of this, such as constantly changing information about the relative risks of the contraceptive pill. At what point does the health educator decide that the evidence is sufficiently convincing that she should begin to educate the public with a new message? If she has insufficient knowledge or experience to judge questions which may be medically or technically complex, how does she decide? Or should she not decide but, rather, discuss the conflicting views with clients and let them decide? Recent controversy over the safety of whooping cough vaccine illustrates the difficulties presented to professionals and the public.[1]

Conflicting Interests

Finally, there are many instances of health education practice where a health educator is likely to find herself in a conflict situation, of which the following are examples:

—when professional judgement conflicts with popular public opinion (such as when the medical and dental profession advise fluoridation, but the public have held meetings and presented petitions opposing it);

—when personal preference conflicts with established policy of statutory services (such as giving contraceptive advice to under-16-year-olds when health authority or local authority policy forbids it);

—when the interests of vocal pressure groups conflict with the established norm of the (probably less vocal) majority (such as anti-abortion pressure groups campaigning to show their materials about abortion in schools);

—when the freedom of the individual conflicts with the interests of the majority (such as compulsory no-smoking which restricts the freedom of the smoker!).

Making Ethical Decisions

We have identified these five areas of ethical concern, and posed difficult questions without providing answers. We have done so because awareness of the dilemmas should lead to greater sensitivity about alternative views, and particularly about the views and rights of the health educator's clients. Secondly, an ethical position is a personal one, and needs to be worked out by each individual health worker. The following questions may help the health educator to think through some of the dilemmas she faces, and make decisions about ethical questions.[2]

1 Do you regard your clients as equals? Do you take notice of your clients needs and wants? Do you believe that your clients have rights equal to your own? Do you genuinely feel a respect for your clients?

2 Do you honestly think you know and understand the feelings of yourself and your client(s)? Do you know what their interests are?

3 Do you know all the hard facts relevant to the decision you have to make? Or is your judgement based on other people's views and second-hand information?

4 Are you able and ready to translate your feelings and knowledge into action? Do you have the skills of listening, talking and taking action as required?

5 Are you able to state why you have taken a decision, giving clear reasons which you sincerely believe (as opposed to decisions made for reasons like guilt or conformity with other people)?

The following exercise is designed to help the reader to consider the ethical issues in two case studies of health education practice. Suggestions for further reading are given at the end of the chapter.[3]

Exercise — Ethical aspects of health education

Case A

The DHSS has issued a circular to all health authorities stating that whooping cough has reached "epidemic proportions", and urging an immediate campaign aimed at improving the uptake of whooping cough vaccination.

The district medical officer is conscious that local vaccination rates are not very high and he is in favour of running a campaign as a priority "to persuade

continued on next page

continued

parents to have their children vaccinated'', using leaflets, posters and films which embody a strong pro-vaccination message.

The secretary of the Community Health Council (CHC), who claims to represent the consumer's view, has expressed opposition to the proposed campaign. She has recently been involved in a case of a local parent who claims that her child was brain damaged by whooping cough vaccine, and she reports that the CHC's view is that a local campaign would induce guilt and stress in parents by bringing pressure on them to take responsibility for risking brain damage caused by vaccine. She also objects to the pro-vaccination publicity materials, which she feels present a one-sided picture, underemphasising the risks involved.

The health district has a health education officer (HEO), whose job it would be to organise the proposed campaign. The medical officer (to whom the HEO is responsible) asks the HEO to run the campaign; the CHC secretary forcefully expresses her opposition to it.
— Identify the different approaches to health education of the CHC secretary and the medical officer which are implied by their views about the vaccination issue.
— Identify the ethical problems for the HEO.
— What do you think the HEO should do, and why?

Case B

A Catholic comprehensive school is renowned for strong discipline, academic tradition and good exam results.

The school health visitor is very concerned that two girls at the school have recently become pregnant, and that there has been no sex education because the Head Teacher objected to it on the grounds that (a) Catholic parents would object and (b) the school's job is to provide academic education — health education is the parent's responsibility.

However, the Head is also concerned about the pregnancies, and under pressure from the health visitor he has rather reluctantly invited her to a meeting of the Parent-Teacher Association to explore the possibility of starting sex education programmes.

The health visitor, who knows many of the families in the area, believes that most parents would be happy for their children to have sex education at school. But she also believes that a very vocal minority of parents (who will probably dominate the meeting) will object strongly, even if the programmes are made voluntary, as they feel it would undermine the academic and Catholic ethos of the school, and encourage sexual experimentation.
— Identify the ethical issues in this situation.
— What do you think the head should do, and why?
— What do you think the health visitor should do, and why?

Notes, References and Further Reading

1   For further reading on whooping cough vaccination, see:

Perkins E (1982) *Decision-making: the Whooping Cough Dilemma.* Nottingham Practical Papers in Health Education No 8, Nottingham and Bassetlaw Health Education Unit, Huntingdon House, Huntingdon Street, Nottingham, MG1 3LZ

2 Wilson J (1970) *Moral Thinking.* London: Heinemann, p 65
   The application of Wilson's ideas on sex education is discussed in:
   Dallas D (1972) *Sex Education in School and Society.* NFER

3 For further reading on ethics in health education, see:
   Campbell A V (1976) Health and human freedom. *J Inst Hlth Educ,* **14** (3)
   Campbell A V & Higgs R (1982) *In That Case.* London: Darton, Longman &
     Todd
   McPhail P (1976) The Moral Implications of School Health Education *J Inst Hlth
     Educ,* **14** (3)
   Williams G & Aspin A (1981) The philosophy of health education related to
     schools. In Cowley J, David K & Williams T *Health Education in Schools.*
     London: Harper & Row, Ch 2
   Wilson M (1976) Health Enhancement or Disease Eradication: some ethical
     considerations. *J Inst Hlth Educ,* **14** (3)
   See also the codes of professional conduct produced by the various professional
   associations.

PART II

PLANNING

Chapter 5
Identifying Health Educators and their Roles

Summary

The major agents and agencies of health education are described, including government departments, the Health Education Council, the NHS, local government and many others. The role of health professionals in health education is then discussed in more detail, and analysed in an exercise. The chapter ends with suggestions and an exercise on improving the health education role of health professionals.

It is obvious that, to some extent, everyone is a health educator, because we all at some time or another have discussed questions of health with somebody else. This may happen very informally, such as when friends or neighbours are discussing their own experiences. Or, health education may occur incidentally through reading a magazine article or watching a television programme. In this sense, everyone may be a giver or receiver of health education, and the informal, unplanned sources of health education are very significant.

Our aim here, however, is to identify the agents and agencies through which planned, deliberate programmes and policies are channelled.

Agents and Agencies of Health Education

The "map" in Figure 1 indicates the most important agents and agencies of health education. Health professionals are clearly important, but it is also essential to realize that there are many other significant health educators who may have an influence on their clients.

Government Departments

Government departments, particularly the Department of Health and Social Security, but also the Department of Education and Science, the Department of the Environment, and the Ministry of Agriculture, Fisheries and Food, have an interest in, and responsibility for, health education in terms of general policy, and sometimes for specific issues such as a vaccination campaign or public information about food labelling.

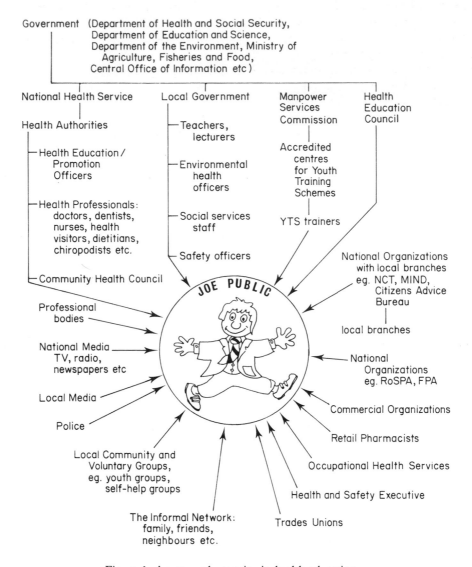

Figure 1. Agents and agencies in health education.

The Central Office of Information has a role in providing information on matters of public health and safety, such as the regular Christmas "don't drink and drive" campaigns. The Manpower Services Commission has national responsibility for the provision of training schemes for young people, which includes "life and social skills" training. The contribution of health education to these programmes is currently (1984) being investigated.[1]

The Health Education Council

The Health Education Council is a government-funded organisation set up in 1968 to promote health education in England, Wales and Northern Ireland. It is a QUANGO (quasi-autonomous non-governmental organisation), and the extent to which its activities are initiated or constrained by political considerations is contentious.[2]
The major activities of the Health Education Council include:
— mounting national and regional campaigns and programmes;
— producing leaflets and posters;
— funding research;
— providing information and resources for health educators;
— initiating and supporting education and training courses, conferences and seminars.[3]

A comparable organisation in Scotland is the Scottish Health Education Group.[4]

The National Health Service

The NHS is concerned with health education, but it is arguable that, in reality, it is a national *illness* service which does not give prevention and health education the priority they deserve.[5]

In the 1982 re-organisation of the NHS, the day-to-day responsibility for health education was given to district health authorities, although in some parts of the country regional health authorities also play a significant part. Some regions and districts have recently developed multi-disciplinary teams which play a leading part in developing policies and plans. For example, Wessex Regional Health Authority has a Positive Health Team.[6] Some district health authorities have "health promotion teams", which may include representatives from local authority departments, such as social services, education and environmental health, as well as health professionals.

Health education officers or health promotion officers are employed by most district health authorities, and are responsible to the district medical officer. Their task is to promote health education within their health district. The numbers employed, and the nature of their jobs, vary widely, but in general their remit includes:
— co-ordination of health education programmes within the district;
— provision of advice, support and training for health professionals and other health educators;
— provision of teaching materials, leaflets and posters,
— working with local mass media;
— initiating policies and programmes designed to promote the health of the population.

Health professionals obviously play a major role in health education, and this is looked at in detail in the next section of this chapter *(the role of health professionals in health education)*.

Community Health Council members may also have health education as part of their work with patients and clients. They can also be an important influence on district health authority policies and plans.

Local Government

The local education authority has responsibility for health education in schools and colleges through the work of teachers and lecturers. There have been considerable developments in school health education in the last decade: many major curriculum development projects have taken place, resulting in significant progress.[7]

Environmental health officers have a responsibility for health education in areas such as air and water pollution, noise, home safety and food hygiene.[8]

Social services staff, including social workers, people working in residential institutions and home helps, are often concerned with improving the health of clients.

National Organisations

There are many national organisations concerned with health education, some of which have regional and/or local branches. Examples of organisations that have no local network are the Royal Society for the Prevention of Accidents (RoSPA), the Teachers' Advisory Centre for Alcohol and Drug Education (TACADE) and the Family Planning Association (FPA). Organisations that have local branches include the National Childbirth Trust (NCT), the National Association for Mental Health (MIND) and the Citizens Advice Bureaux. Most of these organisations produce educational materials and run training courses for professionals and/or the public.

The Mass Media

Health education is also undertaken by national and local mass media, such as television, radio, newspapers and magazines. This is discussed in detail in Chapter 15.

Commercial Organisations

Many commercial organisations have a health education role, by producing educational materials such as leaflets and films, or by providing a consumer advisory service. Manufacturers of babywear and baby foods, safety equipment and drugs are examples. Obviously, health education activity is geared towards good public relations and product sales.

Retail Pharmacists

Retail pharmacists are unique among health professionals because they are so readily accessible to the general public for advice and information in the informal atmosphere of the local chemist's shop.

Occupational Health Services

These services exist in many public and private organisations, including the NHS. Health education may be part of the job of the staff in such services.

The Health and Safety Executive

The Health and Safety Executive play a health education role related to the implementation of the Health and Safety at Work Act.

Trades Unions

Trades unions can be influential in developing health-promoting policies in the workplace.[9]

Professional Bodies

Some professional organisations, such as the British Medical Association, the Royal College of General Practitioners, and the British Dietetic Association, are influential in the policy-making, practice and training of their members in health education. They may also produce educational materials for the public.

Local Voluntary and Community Groups

A huge range of local voluntary and community groups exist, many of which undertake educational work on health matters. Patients associations, self-help groups and youth groups are just a few examples (community work in health education is discussed in Chapter 14).

Other Specialists

There are numerous other people who specialize in health education on a particular topic. For example, some local authorities employ home safety officers, and some coastguards undertake water safety education. Local authority employees in leisure, recreation and town planning departments are likely to have health education aspects to their jobs. Police officers with special responsibility for community relations may, for example, undertake teaching about road safety, alcohol and drugs.

The Informal Network

Finally, as we mentioned in the opening paragraph of this chapter, it is essential to remember that the whole informal network of family, friends, and neighbours is of great significance in shaping people's health beliefs and behaviour; this network is sometimes referred to as the "lay referral system".[10]

The Role of Health Professionals in Health Education

Over the last decade many reports have contained statements in support of an increased role for health professionals in health education,[11] and there have been several studies of the health education roles of doctors, nurses and others.[12] In the introduction to this book we stated that all health professionals are health educators, although they may not separate this element from the rest of their work (such as treatment, therapy and patient care) and label it "health education". The following exercise is designed to help health professionals to recognize the health education elements which are integrated into all kinds of every day work.

Exercise — Clarifying your Role as a Health Educator

The following is a list of types of activity you may undertake as part of your job *which may have an educational element.* (We have excluded many other types of activity — such as administration — which do *not* have an educational element.)

Teaching clients	Working with groups
Caring	Giving therapy
Giving treatment	Counselling
Supporting	Advising
Inspecting	Assessing
Planning	Evaluating
Referring	Working with colleagues
Teaching students/colleagues	

1. Add any other activities with a health education element which are important in your job.
2. Tick the activities you undertake.
3. Identify the educational aspects of each of these activities, giving examples.

(For example, if you ticked "treatment", an example could be "giving an injection". The educational aspects of giving an injection could lie in explaining why it is necessary, what you are doing and what it will feel like. Or, if you ticked "inspecting", an example could be inspecting food hygiene practices in a restaurant, the education aspects might be explaining why the inspection is necessary, what you are looking for, and what the possible consequences of the inspection report may be for the restaurateur. You will probably also tick "advising", since educating the restaurateur about food hygiene practices is likely to follow the inspection.)

Lack of identification of the health education element of a health professional's work is one reason why it fails to be accorded high priority. Other reasons are explored in the next section.

Improving the Health Education Role

A number of factors affect the development of the health education role of health professionals. The need for improved training is recognized.[13] One of the difficulties this raises is how to fit more into the already overcrowded curriculum of basic professional training courses. Partial solutions to this problem might be to review priorities in basic training, and to emphasize post-basic education, such as Health Education Certificate courses.[14]

A problem for students is that they use trained professionals as role models, but research shows that trained professionals themselves may not have the necessary skills.[15] Both health professionals and their tutors may lack an adequate knowledge base for health education.[16]

Some health professionals have too narrow a concept of what is meant by health education, believing, for example, that it means only formal teaching, and may therefore fail to take advantage of opportunities for using alternative methods. Furthermore, the health education needs of the health professionals themselves may not have been met. Although they may be exhorted to set a good example they are often not given the help they need to make health choices and to carry these through. A further constraint may be imposed by the way in which daily work is monitored. There may be pressure to score high numbers of treatments or visits; time spent on establishing a good relationship with clients, and doing an effective job of health education may appear as time wasted.[17]

In summary, the health education role of health professionals could be considerably improved if more emphasis were given to health education during basic training by tutors who themselves had better understanding of health education. Secondly, the support of the health professionals' managers in the field is essential. Finally, a flexible, multi-disciplinary approach to work, with the emphasis on prevention and quality rather than treatment and quantity, would create a climate conducive to effective health education practice.

Exercise — What helps and hinders your health education work?

This is a force-field analysis exercise. It is designed to help you to identify helping and hindering forces in your own situation.

In a stable system, the forces for producing changes are equally offset by forces opposed to change. It is essential to pinpoint all the possible helping and hindering forces, so that you can take steps to increase the power of helping forces. This disruption of the balance of forces results in progress towards change.

For your own situation:
— make a list of *forces which help you*, and *forces which hinder you*, in your health education work;
— identify *ways of increasing the helping forces*, and *ways of decreasing the hindering forces.*

                      Health
Helping forces ⇉ education ⇇ Hindering forces
                      work

Direction you want to go →

Notes, References and Further Reading

1 A survey of Youth Training Scheme (YTS) personnel sponsored by the Health
   Education Council has led to a two-year action research project, which began in
   April 1984, to examine how to introduce appropriate health education methods and
   material into YTS schemes.

   Project Director: Christine Beele, Lifeskills Associates, 'Ashling', Back Church
      Lane, Leeds LS16 8DN

2 For a political analysis of an HEC campaign, see:

   St George D (1981) Who pulls the strings? *World Med*, 28 November

3 *The Health Education Council*, 78 New Oxford Street, London WC1A 1AH
   Telephone: 01-637 1881

   Further details of the work of the HEC can be found in their annual reports and
   outlines of current programmes. The HEC resources centre, including the library,
   can be used by any health educator.

4 *The Scottish Health Education Group*, Health Education Centre, Woodburn House,
   Canaan Lane, Edinburgh EH10 4SG Telephone: 031-447 8044

5 For a more detailed analysis of this argument, see:

   Draper P, Best G & Dennis J (1976) *Health, Money and the NHS*. Unit for the
      Study of Health Policy, Guy's Hospital Medical School, 8 Newcomen Street,
      London SE1 1YR

6 For a discussion of regional health promotion, with special reference to Wessex,
   see:

   Catford J & Nutbeam D (1983) Promoting health, preventing disease: what should
      the NHS be doing now? *Hlth Educ J*, 42 (1)

   Examples of the work of the Wessex Positive Health Team may be seen in their
   Lifeline Reports published by the Wessex Regional Health Authority, for example:

      No 2 *Prospects for Prevention in Wessex*

      No 3 *Filling Gaps: Dental Health in Wessex*

      No 5 *Smoking Prevention—Operation Smokestop: Smoking Cessation Self-help
         Groups in Wessex*

7 For background reading on the development of school health education, see:

   Sutherland I (1979) Health education, the school system and the young. Chapter 9
      in Sutherland I (ed) *Health Education—Perspectives and Choices*. London:
      George Allen & Unwin

   McCafferty I (1979) Health education in the education system. Chapter 3 in
      Anderson D (ed) *Health Education in Practice*. London: Croom Helm

   Schools Council (1976) *Health Education in Secondary Schools*, Working Paper 57.
      London: Evans/Methuen

   Evans M (1981) *Health Education in Secondary Schools—10 Case Studies*.
      Manchester: TACADE

For in-depth discussion of school health education issues, see:

Cowley J, David K & Williams T (1981) *Health Education in Schools.* London: Harper & Row

Some significant curriculum projects are:

Schools council/Health Education Council Project:

> 5–8-year-olds *All About Me* (1977) London: Nelson
>
> 9–13-year-olds *Think Well.* (1977) London: Nelson
>
> 13–18-year-olds (1982) Forbes
>
> 5–13-year-olds *Fit for Life* (1983) London: Macmillan. Materials adapted for slow-learning children

Health Education Council *My Body* project (1983) London: Heinemann, for the upper primary age range. The materials focus on the human body and physical health, with particular emphasis on smoking

Baldwin J & Wells H (1979–84) *Active Tutorial Work.* Oxford: Basil Blackwell
Sets of teachers' guides for a five-year programme of tutorial work in secondary schools, covering personal and social education

Hopson B & Scally M (1982) *Lifeskills Teaching Programmes.* Lifeskills Associates, "Ashling", Black Church Lane, Leeds LS16 8DN
Two loose-leaf folders of materials for use in secondary schools. Use.group work extensively and cover topics such as communication, personal relationships, managing negative emotions, coping with unemployment, and stress

Health Education Council (1977) *Living Well Project.* Cambridge University Press
For secondary school pupils, in three parts:

> *And How Are We Feeling Today?* 35 work cards with cartoons and discussion questions on emotions, relationships and physical health
>
> *Who Cares?* A book of dialogues between young people and adults on problems such as class disruption, petty theft, drinking and driving
>
> *Support Group* 35 work cards with photographs, drawings and discussion questions on difficult situations

TACADE (1981) *Free to Choose.* Manchester: TACADE (2 Mount Street, M2 5NG)
Drug education materials for use in secondary schools

TACADE (1984) *Alcohol Education Syllabus.* Manchester: TACADE
Teachers' guide and pupil materials in two parts—11 to 16 years and 16 to 19

8   For a survey of health education provision by environmental health officers, and the implications for training, see:

Bowman D R (1981) Health education as adult education: a survey of local authority provision. *Environmental Hlth*, Sept

9   For further reading on health education in the workplace, see:

Randell J, Wear G & McEwan J (1984) *Health Education in the Workplace.* London: Health Education Council

McEwan J (1979) Health and work. In Sutherland I (ed) *Health Education: Perspectives and Choices.* London: George Allen & Unwin, Ch 7

10   For discussion of the lay referral system, see:

Friedson E (1970) *Profession of Medicine* New York: Dodds Mead & Co.

For further reading on the influence of informal networks on health beliefs and behaviour, see:

Farrell C (1978) *My Mother Said* . . . London: Routledge & Kegan Paul

Blaxter M & Paterson E (1982) *Mothers and Daughters: A Three Generational Study of Health Attitudes and Behaviour.* London: Heinemann

Graham H (1984) *Women, Health and the Family.* Wheatsheaf Books, Ch 11

11   See, for example:

Dyer L E (1983) Address to Association of Community Physiotherapists. *Therapy Weekly*, 23 April

Dyer states, with reference to the role of physiotherapists: "Traditional heavy emphasis on cure should be changed to that of care and support. We should move away from being salvage operators and turn our attention to contributing at primary care level, where prevention has a major importance".

The need for all the members of the primary health care team to be involved in preventive and education work is stated in:

Royal College of General Practitioners (1983) Promoting Prevention. *Occasional Paper* no 22

The DHSS also supports the need for prevention and health education and the role of health professionals as part of community care:

DHSS (1981) *Care in Action: a Handbook of Policies and Priorities for the Health and Personal Social Services in England.* London: HMSO

12   For more discussion on the role of health professionals in health education, see:

Alwyn Smith E (1979) Health education and the National Health Service. In Sutherland I (ed) *Health Education: Perspectives and Choices.* London: George Allen & Unwin, Ch 5

Tones K & Davison L (1979) Health education in the National Health Service. In Anderson D C (ed) *Health Education in Practice.* London: Croom Helm, Ch 2

13   The Health Education Council has funded a number of projects to research and support the role of health professionals as health educators: these include general practitioners, nurses, environmental health officers and members of the professions allied to medicine. For example, a recent report is:

Lyne P A (1984) *Just Repairing the Damage? Health Education and the Professions Allied to Medicine—a Report on a Preliminary Study.* London: Health Education Council

Useful material produced by the Scottish Health Education Group:

Hardy L K (1982) *Health: Self-appraisal—a Manual for Nurse Teachers.* Edinburgh: Scottish Health Education Group

Scottish Health Education Group (1983) *Health Education Inservice Education and Training of District Nurses, Health Visitors and Midwives.* Report of a Working Party of the Nursing Advisory Committee, Scottish Health Education Group.

14 Health Education Certificate courses for health professionals are one-day-a-week, day-release courses lasting for one academic year; there are about 30 of these courses in polytechnics and colleges of further and higher education. For details, write to the Education and Training Division, Health Education Council, 78 New Oxford Street, London WC1A 1AH

15 For example, nurse tutors and trained nurses may not have the skills in assessing health education needs, or in using experiential methods required to teach communication skills. See:

Faulkner A (1984) Health education and nursing, *Nursing Times*, **80** (9), 45–46

16 Research suggests that both nurses and their tutors may have inadequate knowledge of the dangers of smoking. See:

Faulkner A & Ward L (1983) Nurses as health educators in relation to smoking. *Nursing Times*, **79** (15), 47–48

Ward L & Faulkner A (1983) Tutors as health educators. *Nursing Times*, **79** (40), 66–67.

17 NHS/DHSS (1983) *Reports from working groups C and D of the Steering Group on Health Services Information* (the Korner Committee)

Chapter 6
Identifying Health Education Needs and Priorities

Summary

An analysis of the concept of need and discussion on how to identify health education needs is followed by guidelines on assessing health education needs, illustrated by a case-study. The final section, on setting health education priorities, includes exercises on analysing the real-life reasons for health education priorities and on setting priorities.

Identifying needs and priorities in health education is a complex process which takes place at many levels, from global and national to the level of local communities, families, small groups and individuals.

At global, national and regional level, the assessment of health education needs, and the formulation of policies and plans to meet those needs are part of the work of the World Health Organisation, government departments, the Health Education Council, and regional health authorities, among others. At a district health authority level, policy making and planning is undertaken by senior officers such as the District Medical Officer and the District Health Education Officer. Consideration of identifying needs and priorities at these larger-scale levels is necessarily outside the scope of this book, and our concern is with the level of work undertaken by health professionals with individual clients, families, small groups and communities.[1]

A second introductory point which we need to stress is that we are concerned specifically with health *education* needs. These are, of course, one aspect of the health professional's work, along with needs for treatment, care, therapy and so on, which we have discussed in the previous chapter. Our concern is that health education is integrated into total professional practice, and that health education needs and priorities will be assessed as thoroughly and competently as all other aspects of work.

Before looking at how needs may be assessed and priorities decided, it is helpful to consider what may be meant by a *need*.

Concepts of Need

It is useful to think of four kinds of need.[2]

Normative Need

Normative need is need defined by an expert or professional according to her own standards; falling short of those standards means that there is a need. For example, a dietitian may identify a certain level of nutritional knowledge as the desirable standard for her client and she defines a need for nutrition education if her client's knowledge does not reach that standard. This normative need is based on the value judgments of the professional experts, and this may lead to problems. One is that expert opinion may vary over what is the acceptable standard, and the other is that the values and standards of the experts may be different from those of their clients.

Some normative needs are prescribed by law—for example, food hygiene regulations.

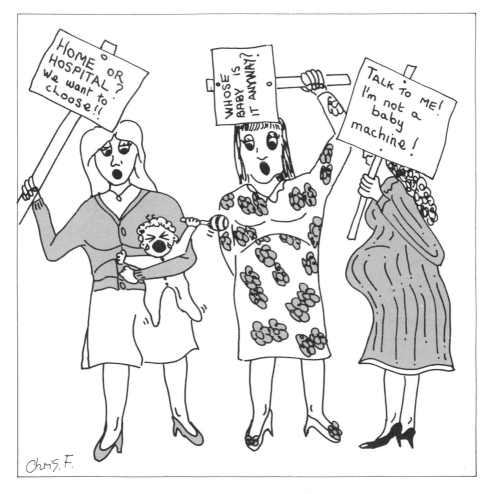

Expressed need is felt need turned into demand!

Felt Need

Felt need is the need which people feel—in other words, it is what they *want*. For example, a pregnant woman may feel the need for education about childbirth. *Felt* needs may be limited or inflated by people's perceptions and knowledge about what could be available.

Expressed Need

Expressed need is what people say they need; in other words, it is felt need which has been turned into an expressed *request* or *demand*. The demand for exercise classes and slimming groups are examples of *expressed* need. It is worth noting that not all *felt* need is automatically turned into *expressed* need. Lack of opportunity, motivation or assertiveness skills could all prevent the expression of a *felt* need.

   Expressed needs may conflict with the professional's *normative* needs. For example, a patient may express a need for a considerable amount of information on his medical condition, and this may be far more than the health professional is able or willing to give. The converse may also happen!

Comparative Need

Comparative need for health education is defined by comparison between similar groups of clients, some of which are in receipt of certain health education and some are not: those who are not are then defined as being in need. For example, if pupils in school A receive health education and pupils in similar school B do not, it could be said that there is a comparative need for health education in School B. This assumes that the needs of the groups receiving the health education are ideally met; this may not be so, as these needs may be over- or under-supplied according to other criteria.

To summarize: *Need, like beauty, is in the eye of the beholder.*[3]

Identifying Health Education Needs

How does a health professional set about identifying the health education needs of her clients?

The Scope

For some health workers, the task has already to some extent been done. For example, a dental hygienist working in a dental surgery with individual patients already has the clearly identified task of educating her patients in oral hygiene. Her next task is to identify and respond to the individual needs of each patient (we discuss the skills required for this in Part III: Practice).

   Other health workers, however, have more choice and scope in the range of health education they can undertake. Community health workers, such as health visitors concerned with preventive health education and health promotion, probably have the greatest scope. The degree of autonomy they have in their professional practice will vary according to the policy of their senior officers, but all will need some skills and knowledge to help them identify the health education needs of their client.

Reactive or Proactive?

It is useful to make an initial distinction between being *reactive* and *proactive* when identifying needs. Being *reactive* means responding (ie. reacting) to the needs and demands which other people make. Pressures from vested interest groups and the media may introduce bias into how needs are perceived, and produce pressure to react. Being *proactive* means taking the initiative and deciding oneself on the area of work to be done and it may include saying "no" to the demands of other people if these do not fit existing policies and priorities.

Being reactive or proactive can be related to the approaches to health education which were discussed in Chapter 3. Using a client-directed approach means being reactive to consumer's expressed needs, whereas using a medical or behaviour change approach may mean being proactive. This is particularly true of preventive medical interventions such as immunization campaigns.

For the health professional, the demand for health education may be anything from zero to overwhelming, and in the latter case she could spend her whole time being reactive. In practice, there is usually a balance to be struck between being reactive and proactive, which brings us back to the central questions: how can needs for health education be identified, and once identified, what criteria can the health professional use to decide whether, and how, to respond?

Health Information

The starting point for defining health education needs is *information* of various kinds from a range of sources. We will now look at the major kinds of health information and how this may help to identify health education needs.

Epidemiological data   Epidemiology is the study of the distribution and determinants of disease in communities; epidemiological data indicates how many people are affected by a health problem, how many people die from a particular health problem (if it is a potentially fatal one), and who are most at risk (eg. men or women? which age groups? which social class? which occupation? which geographical area? fat or thin people? smokers or non-smokers? sedentary or active people?).

Mortality and morbidity data are collected nationally, and some data are also available on a regional and local basis. (Mortality data are concerned with causes of death; morbidity data are concerned with types of illness and disability). Mortality data are derived from death certificates; morbidity data are derived from a wide range of sources, including general practice records, hospital records, sickness absence certificates, child health records, returns of notifiable diseases, disability registration and many others. In addition, surveys such as the General Household Survey, and surveys carried out for research purposes provide a considerable amount of health information.

A detailed discussion of the sources and limitations of epidemiological data is outside the scope of this book, and further reading is suggested.[4] The important point to make here is that epidemiological data provide essential information on the health of the population, the causes and risk-factors related to ill health, and consequently, the potential for prevention and health education.

Social and environmental indicators In addition to the above medical information, there are other kinds of information which may indicate the need for health education. For example, are there problems of housing or employment? Is there a high elderly or one-parent family population? Are there low-income families? What are the social/leisure/recreation/shopping facilities like? Data on these social factors may indicate a need for (for example) education on welfare rights, family planning or getting nutritional value for money. In new work in this field, the emphasis is on developing "positive health indicators".[5]

Professional and public views The views of fellow professionals and the public reflect experience and perceptions accumulated over the years which it would clearly be foolish to ignore. Yet these often are ignored, and health education continues to take place with no real consideration of whether it is really what the consumer wants or is interested in, or whether it accords with the views of the "grass-roots" health professionals.[6]

There are several methods of obtaining the views of health professionals and of the public: these range from informal discussions/interviews to large-scale surveys using questionnaires or in-depth interview techniques.[7]

Key members of the public could include people who have been brought up in the area and are well-known and respected (the opinion leaders), a sample of key clients (eg. mothers), members of voluntary organisations, residents associations, trade unions, or members of the Community Health Council. Key professionals could include GP's, nursing officers, health visitors, district nurses, social workers, teachers, environmental health officers, the police and religious leaders.[8]

Once a particular need for health education has been identified, the next stage is to assess it in more detail.

Assessing Health Education Needs

The assessment of health education needs can be approached systematically by asking a series of key questions, the answers to which will help the professional to decide whether to respond to a particular need, and if so, how.

1 What Sort of Need is it?

Is this a normative, felt, expressed or comparative need?

In a parentcraft class, for example, what kind of need is being met: the *normative* needs decided by the health professional, the *felt* or *expressed* needs of the parents or *comparative* needs decided after looking at what was available elsewhere?

2 Who Decided that there is a Need?

Whose decision is it: the professional's, the consumer's or both?

Sometimes the answer to this question is not immediately obvious, because the need has emerged after discussion between the health professional and client. People do not always know what they need or want, because their awareness and knowledge of the possibilities is limited. It may be part of the professional's job to raise awareness and knowledge of health issues; in this way she may help to create a demand (an *expressed* need) for health education. For example, the public's demand for education about how to stop smoking only came after health professionals had raised awareness of the health hazards of smoking.

The ideal situation is a joint decision by consumers and professionals.

3 What are the Grounds for Deciding that there is a Need?

Is there any evidence of need in the form of hard data—facts and figures? If not, could such data be collected? For example, the case for health education on family planning could be strengthened with data on abortions and unwanted pregnancies.

Have the views of the client(s) been sought? Do they see this as a need? Were the grounds for deciding that this is a need value judgements of a health educator? If so, what values were involved?

4 Is Health Education the Answer to the Need?

Health education cannot solve all problems or meet all health needs; it may not always even be a partial answer. For example, there may be an identified need to encourage women to attend antenatal clinics. Health education messages about attending clinics may be seen to be the answer but in fact may make no difference because the appropriate response is to move the time and place of the clinics so that working mothers without cars are able to attend.

So other ways of meeting the need should be explored, and questions asked whether health education is the most appropriate response, and if there is any evidence to show that it is likely to be effective.

In the following case study, we assess the identified need for health education on the subject of solvent abuse, applying the four assessment questions.

Case study — Assessing health education needs

A problem of solvent abuse[9]

Harry is a probation officer, and aware that the police feel there is a problem of glue-sniffing by teenagers on his patch. The police believe that the other professions are ignoring the problem and have suggested that a police officer should go into local schools to tell the pupils about the dangers of glue-sniffing. Harry talks to one of the local social workers who suggests that a better approach may be to run a group for the teenagers who are sniffing, but she doubts the effectiveness of this.

Harry talks to the head teacher of the local comprehensive school. The head is dubious about the police coming to talk to all the pupils as he feels it may

continued on next page

---

continued

excite curiosity and actually spread the problem. The Head also feels that putting all the solvent abusers together in a group would label them as "problems" and that they would be a bad influence on each other.

Harry also discovers that a group of parents have been lobbying local MPs about the need for more legislation to control solvent abuse.

He finds that there are different views on the seriousness of the problem. The local press sees it as a "deadly epidemic", but the Head feels that most children who experiment do not continue with the habit and that the minority who are chronic users are already known to the school as having a number of other serious problems.

Finally, Harry talks to a group of glue-sniffers about why they do it. They give reasons such as:

— we like it
— to enjoy ourselves and feel "drunk"
— there's nothing else to do round here
— it's better than watching TV
— all my friends do it
— it gets rid of my frustrations
— we're fed up with school
— it proves we can do our own thing

1. What sort of "need" is it?

Only three groups of people have identified glue-sniffing as a definite problem: the police, the group of parents who have been lobbying their MP, and the local press. Of these, only the police have clearly identified a need for education on the dangers of glue-sniffing. This is probably a normative need, based on the police view that everyone should know the dangers and no-one should be sniffing glue. This is their normative standard.

2. Who decided that there is a need?

The professionals — there is no indication that the consumers (the teenagers) felt or expressed any need for health education. Indeed, in their view, glue-sniffing itself is fulfilling a need for an exciting occupation.

3. What are the grounds for deciding that there is a need?

No factual evidence has been cited, but presumably statistics would be available from the police about the numbers of reported incidents, and possibly from GPs and hospitals about patients who became ill or suffered injuries as a result of glue-sniffing. But as glue-sniffing is not a criminal offence, and much of it is likely to be undetected and not result in serious harm, facts and figures are likely to be "guesstimates" at best. Teachers, youth leaders, policemen, social workers, and, of course, the teenagers themselves, could all be asked for their opinions on the size and seriousness of the problem, and whether they feel there is a need for health education.

continued on next page

continued

4. Is health education the answer to the need?

In the light of Harry's discussion with the glue-sniffers, it seems unlikely that the police's idea of educating pupils in school about the dangers of glue-sniffing would have any impact on the glue-sniffers habits. Indeed, the social worker expressed doubt and the Head sees this as counter-productive.

However, health education may have a useful part to play in an overall approach to the problem of solvent abuse. In the long run the most effective strategy could be to look more deeply at the root of the problem, and create more jobs, leisure facilities and out-of-school activities for young people.

A more short-term strategy might be as follows:

Health education directed to:	*Aim:*
Professional fieldworkers	Increase knowledge of solvent abuse, for use when working with young people and their families, especially parents.
School teachers and school nurses	Increase knowledge of current approaches to drug education as part of total health and social education programme for all pupils.
School pupils	Knowledge of use and misuse of all drugs as part of total health and social education programme. Exploration of attitudes and values about drug-taking, role playing decision-making in ''drug situations''.
Shopkeepers	Increase awareness and knowledge of glue sniffing problem. Encourage decision to move glue off display and not to sell it to children.

Exercise — Assessing a health education need

A health visitor is approached by a teacher from a local comprehensive school who reports that a number of girls at the school have become pregnant during the last year. The teacher feels that more sex education for fourth-year girls is needed and asks the health visitor for help.

If you were the health visitor, how would you set about assessing this need? Use the four questions in the preceding case study as a guide.

OR use the four questions to assess a health education need which you have identified in your own work, or one which you are likely to meet.

Setting Health Education Priorities

A health professional may have a huge workload of health education needs which she feels should be met, but there are always constraints on time, resources and energy. Spreading effort a mile wide and an inch deep is probably useless and concentrating effort on priority areas is more effective and rewarding. Before attempting to set priorities it is helpful to analyse current "real life" practice and recognize the wide range of criteria which will affect such decisions.

Exercise — Analysing the "real life" reasons for health education priorities

Identify a health education activity which has a high priority in your work; this could be work which you undertake with a number of clients (eg. antenatal education) or just one (eg. a particular patient); it could be part of your usual work or a special event such as a campaign. (It will be especially helpful for the purposes of this exercise if you can identify an area of work which has recently become a priority.)

Now work through the following tasks.
1. Identify who it was who decided that this work should take priority (eg. you? your seniors? your clients? all three?)
2. List ALL THE POSSIBLE REASONS why this work has priority — include the reasons that you are sure about as well as any that are speculation.
     Your reasons could include any of the following, and probably many more:
     — I feel that it's important
     — it is established policy of senior officers
     — we've always done it and saw no reason to change
     — there was pressure from the public
     — it was in response to a crisis
     — we had to be seen to be doing something
     — there is new evidence of need
     — there is evidence that the work has been effective in a similar area
     — someone has a personal enthusiasm for it (a bee in his bonnet)
     — it was the current national/local theme (eg. the Year of the Disabled or the Year of the Child)
     — we had a new staff member with special expertise which we wanted to use
     — we had to economize and be more efficient
     — it was politically expedient
3. Identify what you think the most important reasons are. Do you think that they are sound reasons for setting priorities?

There can be no watertight method for setting priorities because priorities ultimately depend upon the value-judgements of the professionals involved, but it may be helpful to work through the following checklist.

Exercise — Setting priorities for health education

1. Health issues

Do you define your priorities in terms of:
— health promotion and positive health (eg. ''Look After Yourself''
 programmes[10])?
— health issues (eg. poverty, unemployment, sexism)?
— health problems (eg. heart disease, cancer, dental disease, overweight,
 mental health problems)?
Why?

2. Consumer groups

Who are the people your health education is aimed at:
— policy makers and planners?
— individual clients or patients?
— families?
— selected groups?
— the whole community? If so, how do you define your ''community''?
Why?

3. Age groups

Do you define your priority consumer groups further in terms of age:
— children, young people, young parents, elderly etc?
Why?

4. ''At risk'' groups

Do you define your priority consumer groups further in terms of high-risk
categories, such as smokers, people with high blood pressure, unemployed
people or those living on low incomes?
  If so, why? Have you examined the evidence leading to the identification
of these ''at risk'' groups?

5. Effectiveness

Have you any evidence that health education in your priority areas is likely
to be effective?

6. Feasibility

Is it feasible for you to spend time with your priority group? Do you have
access to this group? Do you have the necessary resources, such as
relevant up-to-date knowledge and teaching materials? Do you have the
necessary skills in health education methods?

7. Working with other people

Do you know what work is already being done with your priority group, by
professionals, community groups and volunteers?

continued on next page

continued

Are you sure that your work will complement any other work which is going on — and not be seen as duplication or interference?

8. Ethics

Are there ethical aspects to your proposed work which you need to consider?
Is your work ethically acceptable to you?
Will it be acceptable to your consumer group?
Will it be congruent with their values?
How may the desired outcome affect their lives?

9. Add anything else which you feel is important to consider

Now identify your *top priority* for health education in your work, and add any other *high priorities*.

Notes, References and Further Reading

1   For further reading on a detailed approach to identifying health education needs and priorities, see:

Green L W, Kreuter M W, Deeds S G & Partridge K B (1980) *Health Education Planning—a Diagnostic Approach*. USA: Mayfield Publishing Company

2   This analysis of the concept of "need" is based on:

Bradshaw J (1972) The concept of social need. *New Society*, 30 March

For further reading on the concept of social need, see:

Forder A (1974) *Concepts in Social Administration: a Framework for Analysis*. London: Routledge & Kegan Paul, Ch 3

For further reading on "need" in the NHS, see:

Cooper M (1975) *Rationing Health Care*. London: Croom Helm.

Culyer A J (1976) *Need and the NHS*. Oxford: Martin Robertson.

3   Cooper M (1975) *Rationing Health Care*. London: Croom Helm, p 20

4   Further reading on epidemiology:

Waters W E & Cliff K S (1983) *Community Medicine: a Textbook for Nurses and Health Visitors*. London: Croom Helm

Barker D J P & Rose G (1979) *Epidemiology in Medical Practice*. Edinburgh: Churchill Livingstone

Donaldson R J & Donaldson L J (1983) *Essential Community Medicine*. Lancaster: MTP Press

McCarthy M (1982) *Epidemiology and Policies for Health Planning*. London: King Edward's Hospital Fund

5   Catford J C (1983) Positive health indicators—towards a new information base for health promotion. *Community Med*, **5** (2)

6   See, for example, the following studies of consumer views on health education:

Adams L (1982) Consumers' views of ante-natal education *Hlth Educ J*, **41** (1)

O'Looney B A & Harding C M (1982) Coronary heart disease: the views of a group at risk. *J Inst Hlth Educ*, **20** (3)

Clarke L (1982) Teenage views of sex education. *Hlth Educ J*, **41** (2)

7   For further information on survey techniques see:

Oppenheim A N (1968) *Questionnaire Design and Attitude Management.* London: Heinemann

8   A useful description and checklist of the kind of health information obtainable about a community can be found in:

Hubley J (1982) Making the community profile. *J Inst Hlth Educ*, **20** (1)

9   Readers interested in the area of drug education are referred to:

Dorn N & Nortoft B (1982) *Facts and Feelings about Drugs but Decisions about Situations.* London: Institute for the Study of Drug Dependence.

Peers I S (1981) *Solvent Abuse—Educational Implications.* Manchester: TACADE

10   The Health Education Council's Look After Yourself programme involves tutor training and adult classes in exercises, relaxation and discussion of health topics. Further details from: "Look After Yourself" Project Centre, Christ Church College, Canterbury, Kent.

Chapter 7
Planning
for Health
Education

Summary

This chapter gives a 9-stage flow chart for planning health education. The stages are: identifying consumers and their characteristics, identifying consumer needs, deciding the goals of the health education, formulating specific objectives, identifying resources, planning the content and method in detail, planning evaluation methods, carrying out the health education, and evaluating the process and the outcome.

It includes exercises on identifying goals and methods in health education, and on planning health education for groups and individuals.

The last two chapters addressed the question of *who* is educating *whom* about *what?* That leaves the important question of *how?* In this chapter we discuss a systematic planning procedure which health educators can apply to their work; it is designed to help them to identify goals and objectives, and to choose the most appropriate methods for achieving their aims and evaluating their work.

The flow chart, Figure 2, identifies the stages of systematic planning and is useful for planning work with communities and groups, and for working with individual clients.[1]

Stage 1: Identify Consumers and their Characteristics

In the previous chapter, we started to consider consumers and their characteristics in the context of setting priorities for health education. (See exercise *Setting Priorities for Health Education*, Chapter 6). The first step is to identify who your health education is aimed at. For example, if your health issue is unemployment, you may identify unemployed people or politicians as the people you want to work with. If your health issue is heart disease, you may identify middle-aged men as your health education consumers.

Characteristics to consider may include:
—numbers: individuals, families, groups, communities;

70

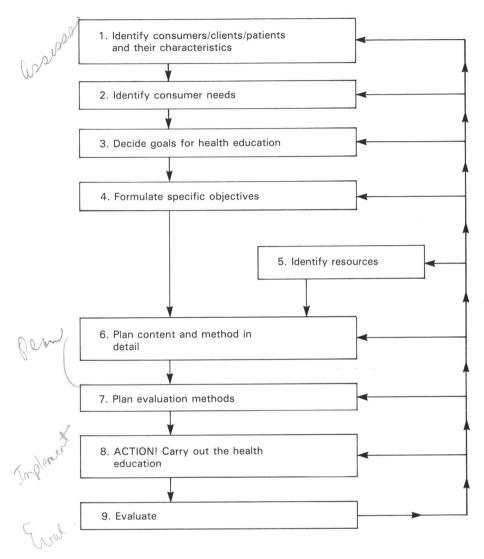

Figure 2. A flowchart for planning health education.

—experience and knowledge of the health issue;
—culture and language;
—attitude and motivation—for example, will consumers welcome your intervention or think it a waste of time;
—expectations and experience in educational methods—some clients, for example, are likely to be frightened away by the prospect of having to participate in group discussion;
—level of ability and receptiveness—for example, are your consumers quick, slow or mentally confused;
—age and sex;
—health problems or handicaps.

Stage 2: Identify Consumer Needs

Again, we addressed this question in Chapter 6, where we identified sources of information for identifying needs:
—epidemiological data;
—social and environmental indicators;
—perceptions of professionals and the public.

We suggested four key questions for the health educator to ask:
—what sort of need is it?
—who decided that there is a need?
—what are the grounds for deciding that there is a need?
—is health education the answer to the need?

Stage 3: Decide on Goals for Health Education

It is helpful at this stage to consider which goal—or goals—you are aiming for. In Chapter 2 we identify a range of health education goals. These are:
—raising health consciousness
—giving clients health knowledge
—improving client self-awareness
—facilitating client attitude change
—helping clients to make decisions
—helping clients to change behaviour
—effecting social changes.

For example, if you are concerned with helping a client to cope better with her baby, the goals involved may be giving the client health knowledge (about what to feed the baby on, for example), helping her to make a decision (about whether to breast feed or bottle feed), helping her to change her behaviour (establish feeding habits) and facilitating an attitude change (so that she changes from feeling guilty that she cannot cope to feeling OK about her ability to be a "good" mother).

Stage 4: Formulate Specific Objectives

Formulating specific objectives is a good discipline because it helps you to think through *precisely* what you hope to achieve; objectives are more specific than the goals discussed in Stage 3.

Types of objectives were discussed in Chapter 2, and three types were identified, concerned with what clients *know*, *feel* and *do*. For example, in the case of the mother learning to cope with feeding her baby, it is possible to identify a precise objective such as "at the end of the session, the client will be able to demonstrate the correct way to make up a feed". If the mother then demonstrates it correctly the health professional will know that the objective has been achieved.

It is less easy to be so precise with other objectives. For example, an objective might be "at the end of the session, the client will be able to say that she feels more confident in her ability to be a good mother". She may indeed say so but there can be no absolute certainty that she really feels it.

But as a rule-of-thumb, we suggest that formulating specific objectives is useful for two reasons. The first reason is that it aids precise thinking and careful planning and the second is that it helps you to evaluate your success. If you can identify an objective which has been achieved, you have a major source of job satisfaction and a basis for further good practice. Conversely, if you can identify an objective which has not been achieved, you know that you need to review and change what you tried to do.

A final point about objectives is the need to make them realistic. The amount of new information, change in attitude, change in behaviour or change in the physical or social environment which can be achieved by one health educator in a limited amount of time is likely to be small, and unrealistically ambitious objectives merely lead to disappointment.

Stage 5: Identify Resources

A number of different kinds of resources can be identified.

The first resource is *you:* your experience, knowledge, skills, enthusiasm, energy and time.

The second resource is *people who can help you.* This may include colleagues who can help you to make your plans, clerical and secretarial staff who can help with administration, and technicians who can help with exhibitions, displays and teaching aids.

The third resource is *your client or client group.* Clients may have knowledge, skills, enthusiasm, energy and time, which can be used and built upon. In a group, clients can share their knowledge and previous experience and in this way help each other to learn and change. An ex-client can be a very valuable resource, too. For example, a successful slimmer, an ex-smoker, an experienced patient or person who has had a particular disease or operation can be a great help to clients who are about to undergo similar experiences.

The fourth resource is *people who influence your client or client group.* This includes clients' relatives, friends, volunteers, patient associations, and self-help groups. It may also be possible to harness the help of significant people in the community who are regarded as opinion-leaders or trend-setters; this group might include political figures, religious leaders or pop stars.

A fifth kind of resource is *existing policies and plans;* for example, if you are planning to do work on smoking, find out if there is already a policy on smoking in your health district. If there is, you can use it to back up the work you plan to do.

The sixth resource is *existing facilities and services.* Find out what facilities already exist and whether these are fully utilized—for example, sports centres offering facilities for exercise and clinics offering facilities for cervical smear tests.

Finally, there are *material resources,* which might include leaflets, posters and display materials or, if you are thinking of undertaking group teaching, rooms, space, seating, heating, lighting, audio-visual aids and equipment.

Stage 6: Plan Content and Method in Detail

This is the stage at which you work out exactly what you are going to do, using the resources available to you. The content will be what you think you need to do in order to achieve the (realistic!) objectives which you have set yourself. Choosing the best methods requires as much consideration as deciding on the content. There is no one "best buy" for health education as a whole. Some factors to consider include:
—which methods are the most appropriate for your objectives (this is explored in more detail below);
—which methods will be acceptable to the consumers;
—which methods you find comfortable to use, bearing in mind that using a new method may feel uncomfortable at first, because of your inexperience and consequent lack of confidence.

HEALTH EDUCATION GOAL	APPROPRIATE METHODS	RELEVANT CHAPTER
Health consciousness	Giving talks Group work Mass media Displays and exhibitions Campaigns	13 11 15 16 14
Knowledge	Giving talks 1-to-1 teaching Displays and exhibitions Written materials Mass media Campaigns	13 13 16 16 15 14

Self-awareness Attitude change Decision-making	Group work
	Strategies for increasing
	  self-awareness,
	  clarifying values,
	  changing attitudes and
	  making decisions
		11
		12

Behaviour change	Group work Strategies for changing behaviour Teaching practical skills Written materials Self-help groups	11 12 13 16 14
Social change	All the above goals and methods applied to the general public and people who make policies and plans about health issues, PLUS lobbying, pressure groups and collective action	11, 12, 13, 14, 15 and 16 14

Figure 3. Guidelines to selecting appropriate health education methods. (These are general guidelines to which there may be exceptions.)

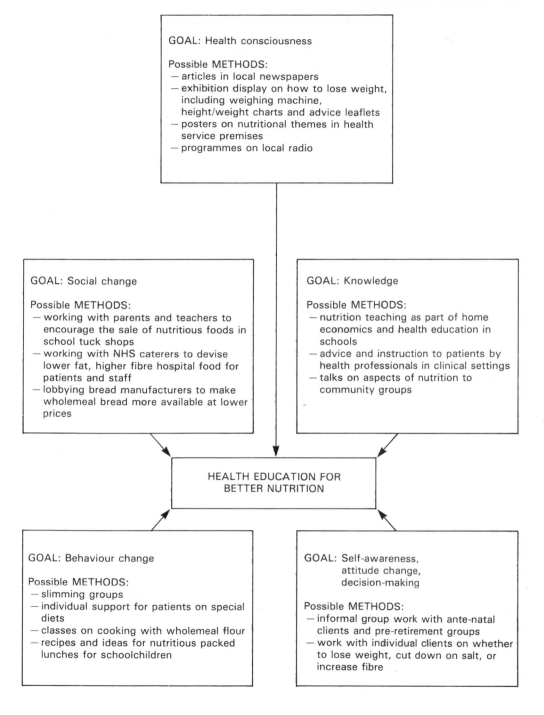

GOAL: Health consciousness

Possible METHODS:
— articles in local newspapers
— exhibition display on how to lose weight,
  including weighing machine,
  height/weight charts and advice leaflets
— posters on nutritional themes in health
  service premises
— programmes on local radio

GOAL: Social change

Possible METHODS:
— working with parents and teachers to
  encourage the sale of nutritious foods in
  school tuck shops
— working with NHS caterers to devise
  lower fat, higher fibre hospital food for
  patients and staff
— lobbying bread manufacturers to make
  wholemeal bread more available at lower
  prices

GOAL: Knowledge

Possible METHODS:
— nutrition teaching as part of home
  economics and health education in
  schools
— advice and instruction to patients by
  health professionals in clinical settings
— talks on aspects of nutrition to
  community groups

HEALTH EDUCATION FOR
BETTER NUTRITION

GOAL: Behaviour change

Possible METHODS:
— slimming groups
— individual support for patients on special
  diets
— classes on cooking with wholemeal flour
— recipes and ideas for nutritious packed
  lunches for schoolchildren

GOAL: Self-awareness,
       attitude change,
       decision-making

Possible METHODS:
— informal group work with ante-natal
  clients and pre-retirement groups
— work with individual clients on whether
  to lose weight, cut down on salt, or
  increase fibre

Figure 4. Goals and methods for nutrition education.

The chart (Figure 3) relates the selection of methods to particular health education goals.[2] (Part III of this book covers the use of these methods and how to develop the necessary skills, and the relevant chapters are listed in the chart.)

It may be appropriate to have more than one goal for your health education, so you may need to use a combination of methods. For example, over a period of time, or even during one session with a group of clients, you may be concerned with giving information and with making decisions, so you could give an illustrated talk followed by informal discussion aimed at encouraging consideration of attitudes, values and decision-making.

The example in Figure 4 shows the range of goals and methods which might be used in a programme of nutrition education. We do not suggest that all of these would be used by a health educator at any one time—they are given here to illustrate the possibilities.

Exercise — Goals and methods in health education

Select a health education topic you are familiar with, such as smoking, exercise, pollution, dental disease, stress, preparation for parenthood or preparation for retirement, and identify the range of goals and the most appropriate methods you could use to work towards your goals.

Stage 7: Plan Evaluation Methods

How will you know whether your health education has been successful? And how will you measure success?[3] These are crucial questions for health educators and there are no easy answers. Large-scale evaluation requires sophisticated research methods, and long-term changes in the health of a population may not be evident for many years, and may not be clearly linked to health education intervention. But modest methods of evaluating the everyday practice of health education can—and should—be used by all health educators.

Evaluation means making a judgement about a health education activity. This judgement can be about the *outcome or effectiveness:* whether you achieved the objectives which you set. So, for example, it could be about whether clients knew how much alcohol would put them "over the limit", or whether clients changed their eating habits and lost weight.

Judgement about health education may also be about the *process:* whether the most appropriate methods were used, and whether the methods were used in the most effective way. For example, evaluating the process of a health education programme could include considering whether it would be better to teach clients together in a group rather than separately as individuals, and assessing the group work or teaching skills of the health educator.

We suggest that you use the following range of methods to evaluate the outcome and the process of health education activities.

Outcome Evaluation

Firstly, consider how you might evaluate the *outcome*. What you assess and how you assess it will depend upon your goals, objectives and methods; we will consider outcome evaluation for different health education goals.

Changes in health consciousness can be assessed by:
—measuring the interest shown by consumers, eg. how many people sent for leaflets, how many people enquired about preventive services such as screening clinics, or educational services such as slimming clubs;
—analysis of media coverage;
—market research using postal questionnaires or street interviews.

Changes in knowledge can be assessed by:
—interviews and discussions involving question-and-answer between health educator and client (to be effective, this needs to be done with skill—see Chapter 10).
—discussion and observation on how clients apply the knowledge to real-life situations and how they solve problems;
—observing how clients demonstrate their knowledge of newly-acquired skills;
—written tests or questionnaires which require clients to answer questions about what they know. The results can be compared with those from a test taken before the health education activity or from a test on a comparable group that has not received the health education.

Changes in self-awareness and attitude can be assessed by:
—observing changes in what clients say and do, during and after the health education activity;
—questionnaires which ask clients to rate their attitudes and values on a rating scale.

Decision-making can be assessed by:
—noting what clients say they propose to do, either verbally during interviews and discussion, or in writing on questionnaires.

Behaviour change can be assessed by:
—observing behaviour of individuals and groups during interviews and discussions;
—client demonstration of new behaviour;
—records of client behaviour. These could be regular records such as numbers attending a family planning clinic or bringing their children for vaccination. It could be a periodical inventory, such a follow-up questionnaire or interview to check on smoking habits six and twelve months after education to stop smoking. Records of client behaviour can be compared with those of comparable groups in other areas, or with national average figures.

Social change can be assessed by:
—policy changes, such as increased introduction of no-smoking areas;
—legislative changes, such as the compulsory wearing of seat belts by motorists;

—changes in the availability of health promoting products, facilities and services, such as the increased availability of wholemeal bread, more free recreational facilities and well-woman clinics.

Process Evaluation

Secondly, consider how you could evaluate the *process:* we suggest three ways.

Self-evaluation—asking yourself "What did I do well in that health education activity? Is there anything I feel dissatisfied about? How could I improve that next time?" Note that we suggest *emphasizing the positive*. It is easy to criticize oneself in a negative, destructive way, which is unhelpful because it erodes confidence. Always look for the positive, and for constructive ways forward.

All aspects of health education can be subjected to this kind of self-evaluation, whether it is a one-to-one session with a client, sessions of group teaching, the production of a leaflet or an interview with a headmaster to look at the health education programme at his school.

Peer-evaluation—asking for feedback from a trusted colleague. Ask for positive comments and for suggestions for improvement. Asking a colleague to "sit in" can be particularly useful for improving teaching and group work skills; it may be helpful to provide your colleague with a checklist of points to look for.

Client evaluation—obtaining feedback on the health education process from the clients themselves. If you are working with an individual client or a group, note their non-verbal behaviour. Do they look interested and alert? Are they looking at you? Are they looking tense, relaxed, puzzled, angry, worried? Some of these factors may not be connected with your performance as a health educator—other factors such as pain and pre-occupation with other things may be affecting your clients—but obvious interest or boredom are clear evidence for the evaluation of your performance.

Note the spontaneous verbal feedback you receive. Do clients ask questions, participate readily, or volunteer any comments about what they got out of the health education activity?

You could also ask for written feedback. You could devise a simple questionnaire which includes questions such as:

Did you enjoy the class/group/exhibition?
Do you feel that you benefited from it?
What did you feel about the way the group activities were run?
Is there anything you would like to have changed?

Stage 8: Action

This is the stage in which you actually *do* the health education, remembering to evaluate the process as you go along.

Stage 9: Evaluate

Carry out any post-activity evaluation you have planned. Use the evaluation to help you plan future health education. On the flow chart (Figure 2) at the beginning of the chapter, there are arrows from the evaluation box back to each of the other stages. This is because your evaluation should help you to re-assess each stage, and plan changes where necessary. For example, things you might want to change could include:

—more concentration on a particular group of clients;
—working on a client need you had overlooked;
—changing your aim of increasing knowledge because you found that clients were already more knowledgable than you had thought;
—scaling down your objectives because they were too ambitious for the time available;
—increasing the use of volunteers and client-support networks;
—making more use of local newspapers;
—changing from giving talks to more informal groupwork methods with clients;
—adding a simple written evaluation form to your repertoire of evaluation methods.

Finally, give other health educators the benefit of your evaluation. Write up your health education projects and their evaluation, and circulate them to colleagues and journals. Circulate your failures as well as your successes, because this may help to prevent successive generations of health educators re-inventing the square wheel.

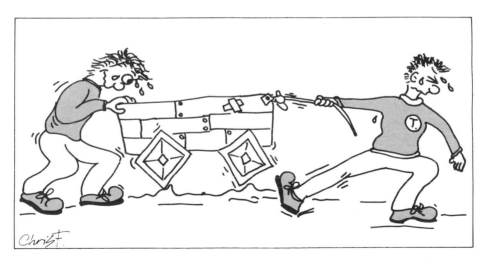

Circulate your failures because this may help to prevent successive generations of health educators re-inventing the square wheel!

Systematic planning may appear tedious and time-consuming at first but, with practice, the stages can be worked through quickly, and it will become an integral part of the health educator's everyday work.

Exercise — Planning health education for groups and individuals

1. Identify a group of clients or patients which you are likely to work with (for example, an antenatal group, a community group, a class of schoolchildren, a youth group, or a group of patients on a hospital ward.) Identify relevant characteristics.
2. Identify what you think their health education needs are in an area where you have the expertise to help.
3. Describe how you would find out what *they* perceive their health education needs to be. (For the purpose of this exercise, imagine that you have already done this, and state what you discovered.)
4. Select one health education need that you have the expertise to help with.
5. Decide on the goals of your health education.
6. Formulate specific objectives.
7. Identify your resources. (For the purpose of this exercise imagine that you have done this, and say what these resources will be.)
8. Write a detailed plan for your health education activity.
9. Write a plan for your evaluation of the process and outcome of your health education activity.

Repeat this exercise, this time for an *individual client.* Select a client or patient whom you know, and go through the stages in relation to the health education you would like to do next time you see him. It does not have to be a lengthy session — it could be a modest 5 or 10 minutes with the client.

Notes, References and Further Reading

1   For further reading on approaches to planning health education, see:

Green L W, Kreuter M W, Deeds S G & Partridge K B (1980) *Health Education Planning—a Diagnostic Approach.* USA: Mayfield Publishing Company. (Chapter 1 gives a concise overview)

Tones B K (1976) *Effectiveness and Efficiency in Health Education.* Edinburgh: Scottish Health Education Group

Tones B K (1979) Past achievement and future success. In Sutherland I (ed) *Health Education—Perspectives and Choices.* London: George Allen & Unwin, Ch 12

Strehlow M S (1983) *Education for Health.* London: Harper & Row, Ch 6

2   Evidence for the effectiveness of different methods for different health education goals can be found in:

Gatherer A (1979) *Is Health Education Effective?* London: Health Education Council

Green L W, Kreuter M W, Deeds S G & Partridge K B (1980) *Health Education Planning—a Diagnostic Approach.* USA: Mayfield Publishing Company, Ch 6

3 For further reading on evaluating health education, see:

Green L W, Kreuter M W, Deeds S G & Partridge K B (1980) *Health Education Planning—a Diagnostic Approach*. USA: Mayfield Publishing Company, Ch 8

Stevens M (1981) Evaluation of health education. In Cowley J, David K & Williams T (eds) *Health Education in Schools*. London: Harper & Row, Ch 17

Sheiham A (1978) Evaluating health education programmes. *Hlth Educ J*, **37** (1)

Green L W (1977) Evaluation and measurement: some dilemmas for health education *Am J Publ Hlth*, **67** (2)

Fink A & Kosecoff J (1978) *An Evaluation Primer*. USA: Sage Publications

Keeley-Robinson Y (1984) *Adult Education Issues for Health Education: a Review and Annotated Bibliography*. Pp 24–30 of Occasional Paper No 1 of the Health Education Council's Health Education Officer Training and Development Study. Institute for Health Studies, University of Hull, Hull HU6 7RX

Parlett M, In Reason P & Rowan J (eds) (1981) *Human Enquiry*. Chichester: John Wiley

PART III

PRACTICE

Chapter 8
Relationships
with Clients

Summary

Educators are invited to explore three fundamental issues: their relationship with their clients, their communication style and the philosophy underlying their educational methods. There are exercises on looking at communication styles and at educational philosophy.

This part of the book is concerned with the *practice* of health education: the skills and methods required to turn philosophies and plans into action. First of all, in this chapter we explore the thoughts and feelings of the health professional about her health educator role. We begin by looking at the relationship between the health educator and her client or client group, and then consider communication styles and educational methods.

Exploring Relationships with Clients

We now ask health professionals to look at some fundamental—and possibly uncomfortable—questions. For example, what is your basic attitude towards your clients? Do you accept them on their own terms or do you judge clients by your own standards? Is your aim to encourage clients to be independent, make their own decisions, take charge of their own behaviour, try to solve their own problems and improve their own coping skills? Or is it to encourage dependency, to solve their problems for them and thereby decrease their own ability and confidence to cope and take responsibility for themselves?[1]

Accepting or Judging?

Accepting people means:
—recognizing that clients' knowledge and beliefs emerge from their life experience, whereas those of health professionals have been modified and extended by professional education and training;
—understanding the knowledge, beliefs, values and standards of the health professional (ie. she understands herself);

—understanding clients' knowledge, beliefs, values and standards from their point of view;

—recognizing that the health professional and her clients differ in their knowledge, beliefs, values and standards;

—recognizing that these differences do *not* imply that the health professional is a person of greater worth than the client.

Judging people means:

—equating a person's intrinsic worth with his knowledge, beliefs, values, standards and behaviour. For example, saying of someone who drinks "People who get drunk are stupid" judges (and condemns) that person, and takes no account of his life experience and cultural background. "Drunkenness can result in people getting hurt" does not judge the client.

—ranking knowledge and behaviour. For example, "I'm the expert so I know better than you" is judgmental; "I know more than you" is not—it is a statement of fact. "My standards are higher than yours" is judgmental; "my standards are different from yours" is not.

(See also the section *Understanding yourself and your clients* in Chapter 9.)

Dependency or Autonomy?

There are a number of ways in which the educator can help the client towards autonomy, such as:

—encouraging the client to make his own decisions, and resisting the urge to make them for him;

—encouraging the client to think things out for himself, even if this takes much longer than simply telling him;

—respecting any unusual ideas he may have.

Autonomy can be hindered if:

—the educator imposes her own solutions to the clients' problem;

—she tells him what to do because he takes too long to work it out for himself;

—she tells him that his ideas are no good and won't work, without giving an adequate explanation or the opportunity to try them out.

We suggest that the appropriate aim is to work towards as much autonomy as possible. Obviously, there are times when a client is dependent on the health professional, and rightly so; for example, he may be ill, confused or likely to put himself or other people in danger. There is also the very real problem that working towards autonomy is time-consuming. However, in the long run, this would be time well spent.

One-way or Two-way Education?

Health education will be a one-way process from educator to clients if:

—she relies on formal teaching methods such as lectures;

—clients are not encouraged to discuss problems and ask questions;
—the educator implies that she does not expect to learn anything from clients (and if she does, keeps it secret!).

Conversely, two-way health education is encouraged if:
—there is an atmosphere of trust and openness between health professional and client, so that clients are not intimidated;
—clients are asked for their views and opinions, which are accepted and respected even if the health educator disagrees with them;
—the health educator tells the client when she learns something from him (eg. "I never thought of it that way before!");
—informal, participative teaching methods are used as much as possible (see section *What is group work?* in Chapter 11).

Health Professionals—The Source of all Health Knowledge?

Health educators deny the value of clients' existing knowledge and experience if:
—they do not find out what clients already know and have experienced;
—information and advice is given exclusively by the health educator;
—it is never suggested that clients can teach and help each other.

On the other hand, the health professional shows that the clients' knowledge and experience is valuable when:
—clients are encouraged to share their knowledge and experience with each other. People do this all the time, of course—knowledge and experience is shared between patients in a hospital ward and by mothers in a baby clinic waiting room—but is this deliberately fostered and encouraged?
—clients are used as teaching resources. For example, experienced parents can be invited to talk to parents-to-be at antenatal sessions, ex-smokers can help other people to give up smoking;
—material is used from lay sources for teaching purposes, eg. television programmes, or articles in popular magazines.

Client's Feelings—Positive or Negative?

A change in people's health knowledge, attitudes and actions will be helped if clients feel good about themselves. It will rarely be helped if they are full of self-doubt, anxiety and guilt. A client is more likely to have negative feelings about himself if:
—the health educator ignores his strengths and concentrates on his weaknesses;
—his efforts are ignored or belittled, even if they are very small or unsuccessful;
—the health educator attempts to motivate her client by raising guilt and anxiety (eg. "if you don't stop smoking you'll damage your baby" or "you're killing yourself with what you eat").

On the other hand, it will help a client to feel better about himself if:
—his progress, achievements, strengths and efforts are praised, however small they are;
—the consequences of "unhealthy" behaviour (eg. smoking) are discussed without implying that the behaviour is morally bad;

—time is spent exploring how to overcome difficulties (eg. practical strategies to help a client to stop smoking). This will help to minimize feelings of helplessness (see Chapter 12 *Helping People to Make Health Choices*).

To sum up, we suggest that health education should be a non-judgmental, two-way process between health professional and clients which builds on clients' existing knowledge and experience, moves them towards autonomy, empowers them to take responsibility for their own health and helps them to feel positive about themselves.[2]

Exploring Communication Styles

The health professional's core attitudes to her clients are likely to be reflected in her style of communication. We identify four basic communication styles: authoritarian, paternalistic, permissive and democratic.[3]

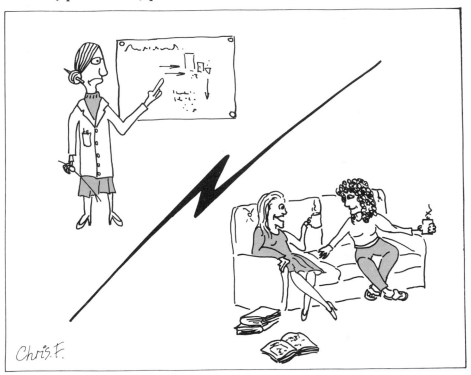

The health professional's core attitudes to her clients are likely to be reflected in her style of communication!

Authoritarian Style

The authoritarian health educator's goal is to obtain strict obedience to her authority, and she relies on her status, credibility and expertise to ensure acceptance of her views. Communication is essentially one-sided, and the client is not encouraged to question or to express what he feels. Situations tend to be seen in clear-cut, black-and-white alternatives.

The positive consequences of this style may be that the client is given clear guidance on how to resolve his problem, and thus feels reassured and secure in his compliant role.

The negative consequences may be that clients are not given responsibility for their own decisions and actions, and that their self-respect and self-motivation may be eroded. Furthermore, clients may respond by rebelling and rejecting the views and decisions of the health educator.

Paternalistic Style

The goal of the paternalistic health educator is to promote the well-being of clients by protecting them from risk. The communication involves mutual exchange: the health educator listens and shows concern for her clients. However, in order to protect clients from the consequences of their actions (eg. smoking), they are made to feel anxious and guilty as a way of getting them to conform and to accept advice.

The positive consequences are that children and vulnerable people (such as the sick and handicapped) are protected from harm and helped to cope—this may influence their personal development positively.

The negative consequences could be that clients become fearful and anxious, reluctant to take independent action. This style also encourages clients to conform to other people's ideas rather than developing their own.

Permissive Style

The goal of the permissive health educator is to let the client come to his own conclusions and do what he wants to do and aims to avoid conflict and to keep the client in a positive frame of mind. Enjoying the educational experience may be seen as more important than achieving specific goals.

The positive consequences are that clients are able to explore their feelings freely and to be creative about finding solutions to their problems. The health educator does not impose her standards, values or opinions on the client, and helps the client to take responsibility for learning.

The negative consequences may be that clients are not allowed to look at uncomfortable issues, and their attention is diverted from their real problems: thus, they may be no nearer to solving their problems than when they began. Information and advice will not be given unless asked for, which could leave clients feeling "in the dark". They may also feel that the health educator is neither supportive nor caring.

Democratic Style

The goal of the health educator here is to use all the resources of her client as well as herself to promote his well-being and to solve his problems. Communication is two-way, with health educator and client listening to each other's point of view.

Alternative actions and their consequences are considered and the cost and benefits of each assessed. Disagreement is not avoided and differences of opinion are aired in an atmosphere of mutual trust and respect.

The positive consequences may be that the client learns to trust his own judgement and at the same time to appreciate other people's rights and opinions. This style also helps people to learn to co-operate and work together with mutual respect and trust, and to make decisions which are right *for them* in the light of available information and ideas.

The negative consequences may well be that strong feelings are uncovered and distress experienced by the client: this may also be distressing for the health educator, and hard for her to cope with (see section *Accepting other people's feelings* in Chapter 10). Also, clients who are used to being told what to do may feel confused and dissatisfied because they are not receiving the advice and direction they want. They will need to have the approach explained to them and be given suitable learning experiences to show them that it works.[4]

We do not suggest that any one style is the right one for all people at all times, but we do believe that the democratic style is most in harmony with the health education philosophy of encouraging and enabling people to take responsibility—both individually and collectively—for health. This style fits best with the educational or client-directed approaches to health education, as discussed in Chapter 3. However, most people have parents who operated one of the other three styles, and many health professionals have been trained by people operating in an authoritarian style; thus, most health professionals are likely to model themselves on what they learnt from their own experience. They are likely to use a medical or behaviour change approach to health education, using an authoritarian or paternalistic style and may need, therefore, to learn how to work in a democratic style—which could be fundamental to their becoming a more effective health educator.

Exercise — Looking at your communication style

The following questions aim to help you to examine your own communication style. Put a tick in the appropriate box.

	Never	Sometimes	Usually	Always
1. Do your clients say what they feel?	☐	☐	☐	☐
2. Do clients finish what they are saying before you respond?	☐	☐	☐	☐

continued on next page

continued

	Never	Sometimes	Usually	Always
3. Do you think you are able to see things from your client's point of view?	☐	☐	☐	☐
4. Do clients disagree with you?	☐	☐	☐	☐
5. Do you explore with your clients the consequences of alternative actions?	☐	☐	☐	☐
6. Do you help clients to discuss painful memories or sensitive issues?	☐	☐	☐	☐
7. Do you share all the information at your disposal?	☐	☐	☐	☐
8. Do you help clients to discover their own strengths?	☐	☐	☐	☐
9. Do you respect your clients' right to reject your advice?	☐	☐	☐	☐

Which communication style — authoritarian, paternalistic, permissive or democratic — do you think you usually use?
What were the influences which led you to develop this style?
Can you identify any advantages in using alternative communication styles in your work?
Can you identify any aspects of your communication style that you would like to change?

Exploring Your Educational Philosophy

The health educator's preferred communication style and her relationship with her clients are likely to be reflected in the educational skills and methods she uses. It is helpful to think of educational skills in terms of a whole range, or spectrum. The factor which changes along the spectrum is the degree to which the educator tries to *control* both the *process* and the *outcome* of the encounter with her clients or group of clients:

Least control ————————————————————————▶ **Most control**

non-directive counselling → discussing → advising → teaching → instructing

(See also section *Who is in charge: professional or client?* in chapter 4.)

At one end of the spectrum comes *counselling*, by which we mean non-directive client-centred counselling where the client decides what the subject of the session will be. The counsellor's role is to listen and to help him to explore and clarify what he feels and what he wants to do. The counsellor does not give advice, state her own opinion or try to control the client's decision. Her role is essentially that of a facilitator rather than a teacher or adviser.

Next along the spectrum comes *discussing*, with individuals or with groups, where the health educator plays a more assertive role. She uses informal, participative educational methods, such as discussion groups or role-play exercises, as ways of helping clients to learn. Clients are actively encouraged to express their own interests, feelings, and opinions, and the health educator may also express hers. Control of the process of the discussion, and of decisions and actions taken as a result, is shared between health educator and clients.

When *advising*, the health educator is trying to control what the client does to a greater extent. This control is not in a physical sense, but happens as a result of the strength and reasoning of her point of view and, perhaps, persuasive arguments.

Next along the spectrum is traditional teaching to individuals or groups of people, such as a community group or a class of schoolchildren. By traditional teaching we mean didactic teaching, such as lecturing, which is firmly structured, centred on the professional's expertise and leaves little or no room for clients to participate. In this case, the educational process is controlled by the teacher, who decides what the content will be, and what she wants the clients to learn.

Finally, there is *instruction:* telling people what to do and how to do it. This is used, for example, when a nurse instructs a patient on how to give himself an injection. In this situation, the health professional is clearly the expert, with the knowledge and skill to pass on to the client. The instructional session is likely to be clearly structured, and the professional controls what she wants the client to do.

Again, it is important to stress that we are not suggesting that any one educational method is always right; the choice depends on the needs and wants of the client, and on the health education goal. As a general rule, we suggest that clients are helped towards self-empowerment when there is maximum interaction between client and professional, and maximum decision-making by the client.

This raises another question for the health educator to consider: why does she prefer a particular educational method? Is it because it is in the best interests of the clients, or could it be that "high control" methods are used because with these she feels most comfortable and secure?

Exercise — You as a health educator

The purpose of this exercise is to help you to focus on your educational philosophy and style and how you feel about yourself as an educator. You can do this exercise alone, but it is better to do it with a partner, taking it in turn to be speaker and listener.

The job of the speaker is to think and speak and, at the end of each section, to summarize her conclusions; the job of the listener is to *listen*, to ask a question if the speaker gets stuck, and to help the speaker to summarize at the end, if she should ask for help.

1. Your educational philosophy

Describe your educational philosophy. Some questions you could ask yourself are:
What do I think my health education is for?
What should clients ideally get out of it?
What is the ideal relationship between me as an educator and my client as a learner?
Do I regard myself primarily as a facilitator (helping people to help themselves) or as a teacher (who provides answers)?

2. Your strengths and weaknesses as an educator

List and describe your strengths and weaknesses. Try to keep a balance between positive and negative. Do this for all kinds of educational methods — counselling, group work, teaching, instructing.

3. How you feel about yourself as a health educator

Try to put into words your feelings about yourself as a health educator. Some questions you could ask yourself are:
How do I feel about myself when I am educating clients?
What kind of educator am I?

4. How do you want to change?

Some questions you could ask yourself are:
Do I want to re-think my attitudes towards clients?
Do I want to learn to use new communication styles?
Do I want to develop my skills in different educational methods?[5]

Notes, References and Further Reading

1   A full exploration of the argument that health professionals undermine people's own ability to cope with ill-health is found in:

Illich I (1977) *Limits to Medicine.* Harmondsworth: Pelican Books

For a shorter account of this argument, see:

Illich I (1978) Medical nemesis. In Tuckett D & Kaufert J *Basic Readings in Medical Sociology.* London: Tavistock Publications, Ch 29

2 For a discussion of the concept of self-empowerment, see:

Hopson B & Scally M (1981) *Lifeskills Teaching*. McGraw Hill, Ch 3

Many of the ideas in this section are adapted from:

Habeshaw T (1983) *Empowering the Learner*. Bristol Polytechnic (unpublished).

See also:

Boud D (ed) (1981) *Developing Student Autonomy in Learning*. London: Kogan Page

3 Based on four styles identified in communication workshops for the parents of adolescents — see:

Brownstone J E & Dye C J (1973) *Communication Workshop for Parents of Adolescents, Leaders Guide*. Champaign, Illinios: Research Press

and also:

Satow A & Evans M (1982) *Working With Groups*. Health Education Council/TACADE joint publication

Satow & Evans identify three basic leadership styles — democratic, authoritarian and laissez-faire, which correspond to three of the four styles we have discussed.

4 Client's dissatisfaction with lack of direction from professionals is illustrated with reference to social work in:

Mayer J & Timms N (1978) Clash in perspective between worker and client. In Tuckett D & Kaufert J. *Basic Readings in Medical Sociology*. London: Tavistock Publications, Ch 11

5 Adapted from teaching materials produced by Sue Habeshaw, Bristol Polytechnic, 1984. Reproduced by permission of Sue Habeshaw

Chapter 9
Some Fundamentals of Communication

Summary

The first section in this chapter is an introduction to transactional analysis as a tool to help health professionals understand themselves and their clients. The next section is concerned with identifying communication barriers, and the final section looks at ways of overcoming language barriers. Each section contains an exercise.

Although everyone communicates, it is true to say that *good* communicators are not born: they are made. Health educators will have learnt communication skills from the people they have lived and worked with all their lives, and probably will have learnt extra skills through their training and professional experience. But self-assessment and development of communication skills needs to be a continuous process, because good communication is fundamental to successful health education, and there is no end-point to understanding oneself and others.

Communication is a huge field of study, worthy of considerably more attention than we are able to give it. We have selected a few key areas in order to identify certain skills and introduce ways of developing those skills. It is only by practising communication and assessing performance that real change can take place; background reading alone is inadequate for developing skills and we recommend all health educators to spend time in experimental work.

We begin with a brief introduction to transactional analysis, which is a useful framework for analysing communication between health educator and client.[1]

Understanding Yourself and Your Clients

An understanding of how people view themselves and their world is very useful for health educators. Everyone has a basic position from which he looks at life, usually largely influenced by his family and the way he was brought up. Transactional analysis theory is a useful tool which can help health professionals to identify four basic positions which they, and their clients, can adopt.

95

"I'm OK—You're OK"

A person adopting this position feels good about himself and confident in his work ("I'm OK"). He will also feel that, in general, other people are trustworthy and basically good ("You're OK"). It is a healthy, optimistic and confident position, operating with a belief that people are equal and have equal worth. However, it does not mean looking at life through rose-coloured spectacles, but accepting that people are basically OK despite their quirks and failings.

"I'm OK—You're not OK"

People who take this position are often critical of others and find themselves putting other people down and blaming them. However, people who like doing things for others also often have this stance ("You're not OK so you need me to look after you"). People like this are likely to have difficulty in learning to trust and rely on others.

"I'm not OK—You're OK"

People with this view will often put themselves down and feel inferior to others. They may feel powerless to change their circumstances and, as a result, get very depressed. People in this position will often discount compliments and praise from other people because "it can't be true because I'm not OK".

"I'm not OK—You're not OK"

People with this view are very vulnerable and may already have health problems such as alcoholism, drug abuse or chronic ill-health. Working with them requires an awareness of how the helper can avoid being manipulated into confirming that "not OK" position, combined with a caring acceptance of the person. It is important to work from the "I'm OK—you're OK" position, treating clients as "OK" equals, in order to start the process of helping them to feel more OK about themselves, more in control of their lives and therefore better able to make health choices.

These positions are based on perceptions of life events and learnt responses to these events. People can re-evaluate events and change responses, and the first stage in this is identifying current life positions.

Exercise — Identifying basic life positions

The four basic life positions are:

continued on next page

continued

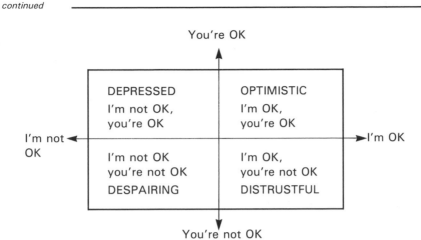

Identify which position each of the following people is most likely to adopt:

1. Peter considers himself to be a good father. He tells his children what they should do and punishes them if they fail to come up to the mark. He expects them always to obey the rules he has set, which he considers reasonable. However, he frequently blames his children for letting him down. His son has recently been involved in a drinking and driving accident. He tells his son that with his upbringing he should have known better.

2. Meg has five children. The health visitor has noticed that although the house is often untidy, the children are happy and often share a joke with their mother. When they are very messy she doesn't get angry, but states openly that it is very difficult for everyone when things get too chaotic, and asks them for ideas about how they can solve the problem — they want to play but everyone has to have space in the house. She listens to their ideas and together they choose the best suggestion for solving the problem.

3. Fred lives alone on a large council estate and has few friends. When people suggest he should get out more he says things like ''But if I visit someone and it isn't convenient for them, I would feel in the way'', ''I can't go to evening classes because I'm not bright enough'', ''I'm not artistic like you'', ''I've never had the luck to have a close friend''. Fred frequently seems to have accidents like chip pans catching fire, and breaking his leg by falling in icy weather. He blames this on fate and moans that no one comes to visit him when he is in hospital.

4. Ann will always help her daughters when they have problems. She says things like ''You poor thing, you can't boil water without burning it. Here, let *me* make the tea'' and ''I'll get this done faster than you can. Let me finish it'' and ''There, there, never mind, everything will be all right. Just let me sort out this mess for you''. Ann worries about her daughters because they never seem to learn how to do things properly, and every time she goes to see them they seem to have some new difficulty.

Using the "I'm OK—You're OK" scheme of analysis can be useful for identifying some of the stances health professionals and clients may adopt. For example, it is easy for the health professional to adopt the "I'm OK—You're not OK" position with clients. One version of this is a "persecutor" position, where clients are blamed or criticized. An example is "Yes, but you don't *try* to remember to take your tablets". A more helpful response would be one where the patient is regarded as OK, such as "What would help you to remember to take your tablets?".

The same position of "I'm OK—You're not OK" may also result in the health professional becoming a "rescuer". "Rescuers" want people to feel better, and to this end they may be falsely reassuring that everything is all right, and try to prevent clients from finding out painful things about their situation. In the long term this is harmful, because it confirms that clients are not OK enough to take responsibility for and control over their lives. For example, a "rescuer" might say "Let me do it for you. It's easy really", whereas a better response might be "What do you find difficult?". Or a "rescuer" might say "There is no need to get upset. Your little boy will grow out of it" whereas it may be more helpful to say "You're obviously upset about this. Would you like to say more about it?".

Clients who adopt the "I'm not OK" position frequently portray themselves as "victims", thus putting a barrier against any help the health professional could offer. For example, a "victim" might say "What do you expect from someone like me— I'm past it at my age". A response which treats this person as "OK" could be "How much do you think you can still manage?". Another example is "I can't do that. I've never been able to manage the baby. You must think I'm stupid". A helpful response which treats the client as "OK" might be "Let's look first at what you *are* managing OK . . .". In these examples, the health professional encourages the "victim" to focus on what *is* "OK", and what he *can* do, rather than focusing on what is "not OK" which would merely confirm his helpless "victim" position.

We now turn to thinking about the barriers to communication which may exist between health educator and client.

Communication Barriers

Health educators encounter numerous difficulties in communicating with clients. Recognizing that communication barriers exist is the necessary first stage before work can begin on tackling these problems; we hope that readers will see difficulties as challenges to their skill rather than as insurmountable barriers. There are no easy solutions to communication problems, but increased awareness and skill can go a long way towards improving communication with clients.

Six groups of communication barriers have been identified by health professionals and researchers.[2]

Social and Cultural Gap between Educator and Client

A number of factors can cause this gap, among which are:
—a different ethnic background;
—a different social class, which may be apparent in dress, language or accent;

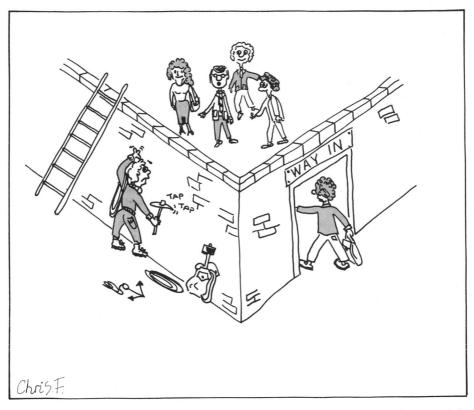

Recognition of communication barriers is the necessary first stage before work can begin!

—different cultural or religious beliefs, for example, about hygiene, nutrition or
   contraception;
—different values;
—different sex.

Limited Receptiveness of Client

A health educator may want to communicate with a client, but the reverse is not
always true, and a client may be unreceptive to a health professional for many reasons,
including:
—mental handicap or confusion;
—illness, tiredness or pain;
—emotional distress;
—being too busy, or distracted by other things;
—not valuing himself or his health.

Negative Attitude to the Health Educator

Some clients may be "anti" the health educator, even before they have met. This
may be because:

—the client has had a "bad" previous experience;
—he does not trust "them"—that is, anyone he sees as an authority figure or part of "the establishment";
—the educator sets an example which conflicts with the advice she gives, so the educator loses credibility;
—the health professional is seen as a threat—someone who comes to criticize and pass judgement;
—the client believes he knows it all anyway, and so thinks that seeing the health educator is a waste of time;
—the client is upset or intimidated because he believes he may be given advice which he cannot comply with because of financial or social constraints, or that he will be asked to give up his few pleasures in life;
—the client "does not want to know" what the health professional wishes to discuss—for example, the results of medical tests.

Limited Understanding and Memory

The client may have difficulties because:
—he understands and speaks little or no English;
—he is of limited intelligence and/or education, and may be illiterate;
—the health professional is using medical jargon which he does not understand;
—he has a poor memory and so cannot remember what was discussed previously.

Insufficient Emphasis on Education by the Health Professional

Communication may fail because the health professional does not give sufficient time and attention to the health education aspects of her work. The reasons may be:
—it was given low priority in basic training, so it is given low priority in practice;
—lack of confidence in her own skills and knowledge which may be the result of inadequate training (see the section *Improving the health education role* in Chapter 5);
—the health professional is too busy, and cannot find the time;
—senior professionals see communication as "just talking" and discourage it;
—reluctance to share knowledge with "unqualified" clients.

Contradictory Messages

Communication barriers are erected when the client gets different messages from different people. For example:
—different health professionals say different things;
—family, friends and neighbours contradict the health professional;
—"the experts keep changing their minds" as information is updated.

The chapters in the rest of this book are concerned with developing skills which will help to overcome most of the barriers which have been identified. Firstly, though, we turn to the specific problem of language barriers.

Exercise — Identifying communication barriers

This exercise can be done alone, but it is best done in pairs or small groups so that ideas can be shared.

Consider the six kinds of communication barriers discussed above.

1. How many of them can you identify in your own experience?
2. What other communication barriers can you add to this list?
3. Which communication barriers cause you the most problems?
4. What suggestions can you make for helping to break down communication barriers? (Share examples from your own experience and make additional suggestions.)

Overcoming Language Barriers

Language is only one facet of the gulf which may exist between people of different ethnic backgrounds. The root of many communication problems is racism; this is a huge topic and outside the scope of this book, but we recommend that all health professionals take time to look at their own attitudes towards people of different races and colours, and at racist practices which may exist in their work.[3]

However, learning a few key words and phrases in the client's language may help to bridge the gap. Words such as hello, goodbye, hot, cold, food, baby, money and words for different parts of the body are useful. Help with learning the language may be available from multicultural education centres run by local education authorities.

When faced with a language barrier, there are some useful guidelines which the health professional can follow to help a client with limited English to understand what is being said to him.[4]

1   Speak clearly and slowly, and resist the temptation to raise your voice in an effort to get through.
2   Repeat a sentence if you have not been understood; repeat it using the *same* words. This gives the listener more time to "tune in" and understand, whereas if you use different words you are likely to confuse him by introducing even more words which he does not understand.
3   Keep it simple. Use simple words and sentences. Use active forms of verbs rather than passive forms, so say "The nurse will see you" rather than "You will be seen by the nurse". Do not try to cover too much, and stick to one topic at a time.
4   Say things in a logical sequence, the sequence in which they are going to happen. So say "Eat first, then take the tablet" rather than "Take the tablet after you

eat". If the listener does not understand or notice the word "after", he will take the tablet first, because that is the order in which he heard it.

5   Be careful of idioms. Being "fed up", "popping out" and "spending a penny" may be totally incomprehensible.

6   Do not attempt to speak pidgin English. It does not help people to learn correct English, and may sound patronising.

7   Use pictures, mime and simple written instructions which may be read by the client's relatives or friends who understand written English. Be careful of symbols on written material; ticks and crosses, for example, may not convey an obvious meaning.

8   Check to ensure that you have been understood, but avoid asking closed questions that require a one-word answer, such as "Do you understand?" A reply of "Yes" is no guarantee that the client really *has* understood (see section on *Asking questions and getting feedback* in Chapter 10).

It is also important to be aware that people's command of English may be patchy; they may understand some phrases and familiar topics much better than others. Also, people are likely to speak and understand English less well than usual if they are under stress, for example, by being in an unfamiliar place such as a hospital, meeting strangers, feeling ill, or worrying about a health problem.

The following exercise is designed to improve skill in communicating with people who speak little English.

Exercise — Overcoming language barriers

The following five extracts come from the district nurse's side of a conversation with a patient whose English is very limited.

"Hello — Oh, we are looking brighter today!"

"Have you been visited by the doctor today yet — did he give you a new prescription?"

"I'll see about your insulin after I've seen how your leg's getting on".

"The doctor says you should take one of these tablets three times a day . . . I don't think you understand — I'll say that again . . . We want you to take one of these tablets three times a day . . . Oh dear . . . (louder) . . . DOCTOR SAYS YOU TAKE TABLET THREE TIMES A DAY".

continued on next page

continued

"I'll leave this list of foods for you. There are ticks and crosses on it to show you what you can eat and what you should not eat. Do you understand? Your son can read English, can't he?"

Using the guidelines that have just been described:
— identify what is unhelpful about the way the district nurse speaks to the patient;
— suggest better alternatives.

Notes, References and Further Reading

1   For further reading on transactional analysis, see:

Harris T A (1973) *I'm OK, You're OK*. Harmondsworth: Pan Books

James M & Jongeward D (1978) *Born to Win*. USA: Signet

Jongeward D & Seyer P (1978) *Choosing Success—Human Relationships on the Job*. New York: John Wiley

Berne E (1964) *Games People Play*. Harmondsworth: Penguin Books

2   For further reading on communication, including communication between health professionals and patients, see:

Cohen S A (1981) Patient education—a review of the literature. *J Advanced Nurs*, **6**, 11–18

Bridge W & Macleod Clark J (eds) (1981) *Communication in Nursing Care*. Chichester: H M + M Publishers/John Wiley

Wilson-Barnett J (ed) (1983) *Patient Teaching*. Edinburgh: Churchill Livingstone.

Byrne P S & Long B E L (1976) *Doctors Talking to Patients*. London: HMSO.

College of Health (1984) Anatomy quiz—how much do you know? *Self Hlth*, (2) March

3   The National Extension College and the Health Education Council together estabished in 1982 a 3-year *Training in Health and Race* project, the aim of which is to work towards a health service more responsive to the needs of a multi-racial society, through the provision of training and training materials for health workers. They have produced a checklist for examining local issues: *Providing Effective Health Care in a Multi-racial Society*. Address: Training in Health and Race, 18 Victoria Park Square, Bethnal Green, London E2 9PF.

Other training materials for racism awareness are:

Katz J H (1978) *White Awareness—Handbook for Anti-racism Training*. Norman, USA: University of Oklahoma Press.

Multicultural Support Services Unit: *Recognising Racism*, a tape-slide set with additional material for teachers. Address: Multicultural Support Services Unit, Bordesley Centre, Stratford Road, Birmingham B11 1AR

Further useful reading for health professionals working with people from different ethnic backgrounds:

Rack P (1982) *Race, Culture and Mental Disorder.* London: Tavistock Publications

Wilson A (1978) *Finding a Voice—Asian Women in Britain.* London: Virago Press

Henley A (1979) *Asian Patients in Hospital and at Home.* London: King Edward's Hospital Fund

Ohri A, Manning B & Curco P (eds) (1982) *Community Work and Racism.* London: Routledge & Kegan Paul, in association with the Association of Community Workers.

Mares P (1983) *The Vietnamese in Britain: a Handbook for Health Workers.* National Extension College, 18 Brooklands, Avenue, Cambridge CB2 2HN

4   Material in this section is largely based on:

Henley A (1979) *Asian Patients in Hospital and at Home*, Chapter 12, King Edward's Hospital Fund for London (see also Chapter 14 on the use of interpreters). Reproduced by permission of King Edward's Hospital Fund for London.

Chapter 10
Basic
Communication
Skills

Summary

Six key communication skills are identified and discussed: understanding non-verbal communication, listening, helping people to talk, asking questions and obtaining feedback, accepting other people's feelings, and giving feedback. An exercise is suggested for each skill.

In this chapter, we discuss the key skills which are fundamental to successful communication and are essential in any context: seeing individuals on a one-to-one basis, working with groups of clients, or working with colleagues and other people involved in health education.

These skills will help to develop better communication with clients, but they should not be expected to provide a blueprint for every situation. They are not a substitute for real understanding; they help by enabling the health educator to express thoughts and feelings authentically (see also the sections *Exploring relationships with clients* in Chapter 8, and *Understanding yourself and your clients* in Chapter 9).[1]

Non-verbal Communication

Non-verbal communication includes all the ways by which people communicate with each other except the words they use, and is sometimes called body language. The main categories of non-verbal communication are:

Bodily Contact

Bodily contact is people touching each other, how much they touch, and which parts of the body are in contact. Shaking hands, holding hands, or putting an arm around someone's shoulders, for example, all convey a meaning from one person to another.

Some health professionals—such as nurses—touch patients frequently in the course of giving treatment, whereas others—such as environmental health officers and dietitians—may not touch clients in the usual course of their work. Touching people is surrounded by "rules" dictated by cultural expectations and taboos, and by expectations of "professional distance", which may be barriers to the positive use of touch in communication between health professional and client. For example, a handshake can say "I'm glad to see you—welcome" and touching a distressed client can say "I'm here for you".

Proximity

Proximity is how close people are to each other. Consider the different messages being conveyed to a bed-ridden patient by someone who talks to him from six feet away at the foot of the bed and someone who comes closer and sits on the bed or a chair. However, people vary in the amount of "personal space" they need, and feel uncomfortable when others come too close.

Orientation

How individuals position themselves in relation to other people and objects is known as orientation. A useful example is to consider the messages conveyed by the lay-out of a room where a small group of people are to be taught. Chairs and tables in rows facing the teacher imply that the teacher will do all the talking, whereas chairs placed in a circle without desks or tables to act as barriers imply that teaching will be informal and that everyone will be encouraged to participate.

Level

This refers to differences in height between people. Generally, communication is more comfortable if people are on the same level; so it feels better to bend down to talk to a child, for instance, or to sit down to talk to a patient lying in bed. Talking to someone on a physically different level can leave one or both parties feeling disadvantaged, and sometimes this is done deliberately: not inviting someone to sit down when he enters an office conveys the message that he is not welcome and should leave soon!

Posture

Posture is how people stand, sit or lie. For example, are they upright or slouched, arms crossed or not? Posture can convey a message of tension and anxiety, for example, by being hunched up with arms crossed, or one of welcome by being upright with arms outstretched.

Physical Appearance

All kinds of messages may be conveyed by physical appearance, such as a person's social standing, his personality, tidy habits or concern with fashion. Their physical appearance is very important to health professionals because of the message it conveys to clients. The nurse's uniform may give the message of professional competence and authority, while the social worker in jeans may signal that she is a non-authoritarian friend, there to help by working on an equal footing with the client.

Facial Expression

Facial expression can obviously indicate feelings, such as sadness, happiness, anger, surprise and puzzlement.

Hand Movements and Head Movements

Movements of the hands and head can be very revealing. Nods and shakes of the head obviously convey agreement and disagreement without the need for words. Clenched fists, fidgeting hands (and tapping feet) reveal stress and tension, whereas still, open hands denote a relaxed frame of mind. Mental discomfort, such as confusion or worry, is often shown by putting the hands to the head and playing with the hair, stroking the beard or rubbing the forehead.

Direction of Gaze and Eye Contact

Whether people are "looking each other straight in the eye" is significant. As a general rule, the speaker will look away from the listener for part of the time when speaking, but will maintain direct eye contact occasionally. When the speaker concentrates on what she is saying her eyes will tend to wander, although she is not conscious of this because her mind is on what she is saying. She will look directly at the listener when she wants a response. If she doesn't look at the listener, it may be because she is uncomfortable with the listener, or with what she is saying; for example, it may be very difficult to look a patient straight in the eye when giving him bad news about the results of medical tests. For the listener, the general rule is that he will look at the speaker straight in the eye while he is paying attention to what she says, but will look elsewhere if his attention has wandered. This is important for the health professional: a client who is talking to her will infer that she is not listening if he finds that she is looking elsewhere than at him. This is particularly important for a client in distress, who really needs to feel that the health professional is giving the client her full attention (there is more about the skills of listening later in this chapter).

Non-verbal Aspects of Speech

Consider in how many ways a word like "no" can be said. The way in which it is said can convey meanings such as anger, doubt or surprise. Tone and timing are two non-verbal aspects of speech which convey messages to the listener.

Raised awareness of non-verbal communication can help the health educator to understand her clients better. For example, a client who says "Yes, I understand" in a doubtful tone of voice, with a puzzled frown or with clenched fists clearly requires further help. Words alone are only a part of the message, and can be misleading.

Non-verbal communication is a fascinating area, and worth further study.[2]

Exercise — Non-verbal communication in your work

Work through the following discussion questions and exercises with a partner.

1. When do you touch your patients or clients, if at all? (Do not count occasions when you touch them while giving physical care or treatment). What "rules" govern when it is acceptable/unacceptable to touch them? Would your clients be helped if you were to touch them more often?

2. Carry on a conversation with your partner, at first standing too close for comfort and then standing too far away. What does it feel like? What is the most comfortable distance at which to hold a conversation? What implications does this have for your work?

3. Describe where you place yourself in relation to your client(s) when you undertake health teaching. For example, when you are talking to an individual, where do you sit or stand in relation to him? Is furniture a barrier between you? If you talk to a group of people, how do you prefer to seat them? Do you think communication could be improved by making changes — if so, what changes?

4. Have a conversation with your partner where one of you is sitting and the other is standing. Both describe your feelings. Do you ever talk to or teach clients who are on a physically lower level than you? What are the implications of working with clients on a different physical level?

5. Practice tense and relaxed postures, then welcoming and rejecting postures. Which do you normally adopt with clients?

6. Identify a few colleagues and clients that you know fairly well. Think back to your first impressions of these people. Do you think that your first impressions were right? What were the important features of their appearance which led to your first impression?
    What is the importance of physical appearance in your job? If you wear a uniform, or a white coat, how do you think it affects the relationship between you and your clients?

7. Look around at other people in the room. What can you infer from their facial expressions, their hand movements and their head movements? What is the importance of noticing facial expression, hand and head movements in your job?

8. Hold a conversation with your partner while staring into each other's eyes all the time, and then converse without looking at each other at all; describe your feelings. Watch two people talking. Do they look directly at each other or do they frequently look away? Do they look more at each other when speaking or when listening? How important is eye contact in your job?

9. Say "I don't know" in as many ways as possible, trying to convey a different feeling each time, such as despair, confusion and irritation. How important are the non-verbal aspects of your clients' speech?[3]

Listening

A primary skill needed by the health educator is that of effective listening, in order to help the client to talk and to discover the client's needs.

Listening is an *active* process. It is not the same as merely hearing words. It involves a conscious effort to listen to words, to the way that they are said, to be aware of the feelings shown and of attempts to hide feelings. It means taking note of the non-verbal communication as well as the spoken words. The listener needs to concentrate on giving the speaker her full attention by adopting a non-threatening posture and ensuring that both the speaker and she are on the same level.

It is easy to allow attention to wander. Some of the things that a listener may find herself doing instead of listening include planning what to say next, thinking about a similar experience, interrupting, agreeing or disagreeing, judging, blaming or criticizing, interpreting what the speaker says, thinking about the next job to be done or just plain day-dreaming!

The task of the listener is to help the client to talk about his situation unhurriedly and without interruption, so that she can help him to express his feelings and explore his knowledge, values and attitudes. This reinforces the speaker's responsibility for himself and is essential for helping him towards greater responsibility for his own health choices.

Experience — Learning to listen

Work in groups of from three to six people. Appoint someone as a timekeeper.

1. Person A speaks for two minutes, without interruption, on a subject of her choice to do with work (eg. safety in the home, or keeping fit).
   Everyone else in the group listens, without interrupting or taking notes.

2. Person B repeats as much as she can remember, without anyone else interrupting. B may *not:*
   — add anything extra to what A said;
   — give interpretations (eg. "It's obvious from what she said that . . .");
   — give comments (eg. "She's just like me . . .").

3. A, and the rest of the group, identify what was inaccurate, forgotten or added.

4. Repeat, with different topics, until everyone has had a turn at being A and B.

5. Discuss the following questions:
   What helped me to listen?
   What helped me to remember?
   What hindered my listening?
   What hindered my remembering?
   What did I learn about myself as a listener?

Helping People to Talk

As we have said, the main task of the listener is to help the client to talk. There are several useful techniques.[4]

Giving an Invitation to Talk

To get someone started it may be helpful to give him a specific invitation to talk. Examples are:

"You don't seem to be your usual self today. Is something on your mind?"
"Is there anything you specially want to talk about?"
"You look worried—are you?"

Clients who have difficulty in talking about their personal problems may avoid doing so by discussing less important issues. They may be helped by asking "Is there anything else?" at the end of the conversation.

Giving Attention

This means listening closely to what the client is saying, and being fully aware of all the ways the client is communicating, including his non-verbal behaviour. It requires effort and concentration on the part of the listener, who should be giving the client her full and undivided attention.

Encouraging

This means making the occasional intervention to encourage the client to carry on talking. It tells the client that the listener really *is* listening and wanting to hear what the client is saying. Such interventions include noises like "mm mm", words such as "yes . . ." and short phrases such as "I see . . ." or "And then?" or "Go on . . .".

Another useful intervention is the repetition of a key word which the client has just used. For example, if the client says "My work's getting on top of me", repeat the word "work . . .?"

Paraphrasing

This is a concise response to the client which states the essence of what he is saying in the listener's own words, using key words and phrases—for example, "So you're not sure whether to have the baby vaccinated or not?"

Reflecting Feelings

This involves mirroring back to the client, in verbal statements, the feeling he is communicating. To do this it helps to listen for words about feelings, and to observe body language. For example, "You seem pleased", "You are obviously upset".

Reflecting Meanings

This means joining feelings and content in one succinct response, to get a reflection of meaning:

"You feel . . . because . . ."
"You are . . . because . . ."
"You're . . . about . . ."

For example:
"You feel pleased about your progress"
"You're depressed because your children have grown up and left home"

Summing Up

This is a brief re-statement of the main content and feelings a speaker has expressed throughout a conversation. Check back with the client to ensure that the statement is accurate. "It seems to me that the main things you've been saying are . . . does that cover it?"

Exercise — Helping people to talk

Work in pairs.
Each person chooses a topic she feels strongly about (which might be a personal experience or a topic of general concern such as disarmament, going on strike, cuts in the health service or violence on television). Stay with the same topic for all three stages of the exercise.
(The whole exercise takes about 45 minutes.)

Stage 1 — Giving attention

One person speaks for two minutes, and the other listens, giving only non-verbal feedback. Then swop roles. After both of you have had your turn, spend 10 minutes discussing these questions:
When you were listening:
— what did you find difficult about listening?
— did your mind wander?
— did you maintain eye contact?
— what did you notice about the speaker's non-verbal communication?

When you were speaking:
— what did the listener do which helped you to talk?
— did the listener do anything which made it difficult for you to talk?

Stage 2 — Encouraging

One person speaks for two minutes. The other listens and gives encouraging interventions (such as "mm mm"), words ("yes . . .") and non-directive comments ("I see . . .") or repeats key words. Then swop roles. Then spend five minutes discussing these questions:
When you were listening:
— what sort of interventions did you make?
— how did you feel about making them?

continued on next page

continued

When you were speaking:
— what interventions did you notice?
— did you find them helpful?

Stage 3 — Paraphrasing, reflecting back and summing-up

One person speaks for five minutes and the other listens. The listener makes encouraging interventions as in Stage 2, but *also* paraphrases, reflects feelings and reflects meaning when she feels it is appropriate. At the end, she makes a brief statement summing up the main content and feelings of the speaker, checking with the speaker that her summing-up is accurate.

Then exchange roles, followed by 10 minutes discussing these questions:
When you were listening:
— what sort of interventions did you make?
— how did you feel about making them?

When you were speaking:
— what interventions did you notice?
— did you find them helpful?

Asking Questions and Obtaining Feedback

Skillful questioning will help clients to give clear, full and honest replies. It is useful to distinguish different kinds of questions.

Types of Questions

Closed questions are questions which require short, factual answers, often only one word. Examples are:

"What is your name?"
"Is this address correct?"
"Are you able to come back to the clinic again next Tuesday?"

Closed questions are appropriate when brief, factual information is required. They are not appropriate when the aim is to encourage the client to talk at more length. So "Did you manage to stick to your diet last week?", which could be answered by "yes" or "no", is not the best way to encourage the client to talk about his experience of trying to diet. A better question would be an open question, such as "How did you get on with your diet last week?"

Open questions give an opportunity for full answers. Examples are:

"How did you manage yesterday?"
"How do you feel about going into hospital?"
"What do you think about trying to do these exercises once a day?"

Note that phrases such as 'How do you feel about . . ." and "What do you think about . . ." are useful for encouraging a full response.

Biased questions indicate the answer which the questioner wants to hear, or expects to hear. In other words, biased questions are likely to bias the response by leading the client in a particular direction. Examples are:

"You're feeling better today, aren't you?" (This is biased because it would be easier for the client to say "yes" than "no").
"You *have* been doing what we discussed last time, haven't you?"
"Surely you aren't going to do *that*, are you?"

Multiple questions contain more than one question. Multiple questions are likely to confuse the listener, who will not know which question to answer, and is unlikely to be able to remember all that he was asked. Examples are:

"Is this a serious problem for you—when did it start?"
"Do you think your constipation would improve if you were to eat more fibre—that's roughage—do you know what I mean by "roughage" and which foods it's in?"
"Are you sure you know what to do or would you like me to explain it again?"
"It might help if you were to rest more—do you get a chance to put your feet up during the day and do you sleep all right at night?"

Exercise — Asking questions

Work in groups of about 10 people.
Decide on a topic on which it is easy to think of questions — such as pets, holidays, my job, or my family.
Person A volunteers to answer questions.
Person B observes the length of A's response to questions.
Person C observes A's non-verbal behaviour (body language).
Everyone else has the task of asking questions.

Firstly, everyone, in turn, asks a *closed* question on the topic.
Secondly, everyone in turn asks an *open* question on the topic.
Thirdly, everyone asks *biased* questions on the topic.

After these three rounds of questions:
Person A says how she felt about having to answer the three different kinds of questions (eg. clear? muddled? irritated? angry? confused?).
Person B says what she observed about the length of A's responses to the three kinds of questions.
Person C says what she observed about A's non-verbal behaviour when answering the three different kinds of questions.

Discuss the application of what you found out to your work.

Getting Feedback

After a client has been given some information, or has been taught a skill, it is very important to check to make sure that the client really *has* understood what was said and remembered it, or mastered the skill he was taught. This is especially important when there is some doubt about how much has been understood—for example, because the client has a limited command of English. There are two key points to note about getting feedback.

It is your responsibility to ensure that the client has "got it", so make sure this is conveyed in your questions. For example, say "I'd like to make sure I've explained this properly, so could you please tell me what you're going to do about it tomorrow?" or "I think I might have rushed through this, and as it is rather complicated to understand at first, could you please show me how you would . . ." or "May I check to make sure I've covered everything—could you just recap what you've learnt so far?" Phrased in this way, clients are less likely to "lose face" or feel embarrassed and stupid if they have not understood. The important point is that you take responsibility for successful education, rather than expecting the client to take total responsibility for successful learning, which would be implied if you asked a question such as "Let's see if you've learnt how to do it properly—could you show me?"

Ask open questions. Closed questions such as "Do you understand?" are not an adequate way of getting feedback. A client may answer "yes" because he is embarrassed, intimidated or afraid of making a fool of himself by admitting that he does not understand. Or he might just want to draw the conversation to a quick conclusion. Ask open questions, such as those in the paragraph above "Could you please tell me what you're going to do . . .", "Show me how you would . . .", or "Could you just recap . . .".

In an informal group, it may be possible to ask an open question such as "I'm interested in knowing what you've got from this afternoon's session—would you like to tell me what was most useful to you?" Success with this method will depend on knowing the group well, otherwise it could lead to an embarrassed silence or white lies to keep you happy!

Accepting Other People's Feelings

The health professional's response to her client's feelings are of critical importance to the client. The best response is one which helps the client to talk openly, trusting the health professional to be an honest and supportive listener who will respect confidentiality where appropriate. This is especially important when the client is talking about something very personal or distressing, or any matter which he finds hard to talk about.

Supposing, for example, a client who is looking tense, worried and near to tears says: "I'm really worried that I won't be able to cope".

A *helpful* response shows that the health professional accepts that the client is feeling distressed and that she is prepared to listen to him as he expresses his feelings and talks about what distresses him. She will then be able to help him by responding to any requests he may make for support, information or advice.

Helpful responses could be:

"What worries you most?"	—an open question encouraging him to express his fears.
"You seem upset about this"	—reflecting back the feeling, showing acceptance of the client's distress and encouraging him to talk more about it.
"You're worried? You feel you won't be able to cope?"	—both these statements repeat key words, showing acceptance and encouraging the client to say more.

An *unhelpful* response is one which attempts to get the client to bottle up his feelings and deny that he is distressed. Other unhelpful responses include jumping in prematurely with advice, or shifting attention to something else. It is also possible to trivialize the cause of the distress, causing the client to feel put down or rejected.

Unhelpful responses might be:

"Don't worry—you'll find you can cope"	—This discourages the client from expressing and exploring his worries. Saying "don't worry" or "never mind" or similar phrases are common responses to people in distress. A principle reason is that an open display of distress causes potential helpers to feel distressed too. So attempting to bottle up the distress with premature reassurance and sympathetic soothing is a way out for the helper who cannot cope with her own distress, let alone her client's.
"Lots of people feel that way at first"	—This diverts attention from the client, who is concerned about *himself*, not with other people.
"You don't need to upset yourself" or "You worry too much"	—This is a put-down, as it implies that the worry is trivial and unnecessary.
"What I think you should do is . . ."	—Premature advice has stopped the client from exploring his worries, while the health professional has leapt in having already decided (perhaps wrongly) that she understands the problem. This has the effect of making the health professional feel better because she feels she has done something positive and constructive. It is possible, too, that the client feels better at the prospect of being able to do something because he has been given constructive guidance. However, the danger is that the client may only feel better in the short term, because his basic problems have not been addressed, and will surface again later. It is essential to spend time exploring the problem thoroughly in the first instance.

"I expect you will   —This is patronizing, and discourages the client from first
have difficulty, but we're   fully exploring ways to help himself.
all here to help you"

Exercise — Acceptance and denial of other people's feelings

Imagine that you are seeing a patient or client who has a problem; specify
what the problem is (eg. he has to have an operation, his marriage is breaking
up, or he has just lost his job). He looks tense and tired. He says "I'm at my
wits' end".

List all the possible initial responses that you could make — including both
helpful and unhelpful responses.

Now go through your list of responses, and discuss which ones could be
helpful and accept the client's feelings, and which are unhelpful and deny the
client's feelings. Identify the reasons for saying that the responses are helpful
or unhelpful.

Giving Feedback

Giving feedback is an important part of any educational process. As with other aspects
of communication, there are helpful and less-helpful ways of doing it.

Positive Feedback

Giving positive feedback is a pleasure for both educator and client, but it is easy
to overlook when concentrating on what still needs to be learnt or improved. It can
make a world of difference to a client if he hears:

"When I remember what you were like three weeks ago, I can see that you've made
tremendous progress . . ."
"I think you coped really well yesterday . . ."
"I feel that you've been making a big effort".

Negative Feedback

Giving negative feedback is less easy, but necessary at times. Negative feedback may
be required when a client needs to be corrected or challenged. We suggest some
principles which may help the health professional to give negative feedback in a caring,
supportive way.

Emphasize the positive: try to balance negative feedback with positive feedback.
For example, say "I know you're still finding it difficult to cut down on the cigarettes,
but you are doing well with cutting down on fat and salt in your food".

It is also much more positive and encouraging to say "You're nearly right" rather
than "You're wrong". For example, say "Good—that's almost right, all you need
to remember as well is to . . ." rather than "No, that's not right, you've forgotten
to . . .".

Challenging Feedback

Sometimes the health professional may wish to challenge the client about his attitudes, beliefs or behaviour. This can be uncomfortable for some health professionals who are not used to being assertive; a useful way is to think about the process in stages.[5]

The first stage is to make an objective statement about the client's behaviour ("You have avoided talking about how much you drink"). The second stage is to say what the effect of this is on you ("This makes me feel that you don't want to face up to it"). The third stage is to make a request for a change ("I'd like us to talk about it"), and the fourth stage is to invite the client to comment ("What do you feel about it?"). This is clear, and non-aggressive but it challenges the client.

Another example is: "You haven't mentioned going for another smear test although you are due to have one. It seems to me that you want to put it out of your mind. I would like you to consider going for another one. What do you think?"

Exercise — Giving Challenging Feedback

Work out what you could say in each of the following situations, using the four-stage process:

1. Make an objective statement about the behaviour or attitude which concerns you;
2. Say what effect this has on you;
3. Make a request for a change;
4. Invite the other person to comment.

In each case, say out loud to a partner what you plan to say in the following situations:

A. You are a visiting speaker to a class of 14-year-olds in a school. A group in the corner are messing around and distracting the others. You want to confront this group with their disruptive behaviour.
B. You are an environmental health officer. You have repeatedly advised the owner of a cafe that he needs to improve the hygiene in his kitchen. You are exasperated because he has taken no notice. You want to give him a last chance to improve and if he does not, you will start legal proceedings.
C. You are a GP. You have a patient who is a heavy smoker with chronic bronchitis. He refuses to believe that smoking aggravates his condition; he believes his chestiness is due to "fate", over which he has no control. You want to confront him with the fact that cutting down on smoking could help his health.
D. You feel annoyed with a colleague who thinks that the effort you put into health education is a waste of time. You want to challenge his view.
E. You are a dietitian. You have an overweight patient who returns to the outpatient clinic every few weeks, without having lost weight or apparently having tried to do so. You want to confront him with the fact

continued on next page

continued

> that giving him yet another follow-up appointment will be wasting your time and his.
>
> Identify situations in your work where you want to challenge someone. What could you say?

Notes, References and Further Reading

1 For further reading on communication skills, including counselling and assertiveness skills, see:

Bolton R (1979) *People Skills.* Englewood Cliffs, NJ: Prentice-Hall

Munro E A, Manthei J J & Small J J (1979) *Counselling: a Skills Approach.* Wellington, New Zealand: Methuen

Egan G (1981) *The Skilled Helper.* California: Brooks-Cole

Nurse G (1980) *Counselling and the Nurse.* Chichester: H M + M Publishers/John Wiley

Nurse G (1983) Counselling. In Clark J & Henderson J (eds) *Community Health.* Edinburgh: Churchill Livingstone, Ch 28

Stanton N (1982) *What Do You Mean—'Communication'?* Harmondsworth: Pan Books

(This book is about communication in the business world, but much of it is relevant to health professionals.)

Turner C (1983) *Developing Interpersonal Skills*, Management in College Series, published by The Further Education Staff College, Coombe Lodge, Blagdon, Bristol BS18 6RG

(This book is intended for staff in further education colleges who wish to develop interpersonal skills, but it is also useful for health professionals.)

Smith M (1975) *When I Say No, I Feel Guilty.* New York: Dial Press. (On assertiveness.)

Dickson A (1982) *A Woman in Your Own Right.* London: Quartet Books. (On assertiveness for women.)

2 For further reading on non-verbal communication, see: Argyle M (1975) *Bodily Communication.* London: Methuen

Morris D (1977) *Manwatching.* London: Triad/Panther

3 Adapted from teaching materials produced by Sue Habeshaw, Bristol Polytechnic Reproduced by permission of Sue Habeshaw

4 See: Bolton, R. (1979). *People Skills.* Englewood Cliffs NJ: Prentice Hall, Chs 3 & 4

5 This analysis is adapted from:

Turner C (1983) *Developing Interpersonal Skills*, Ch 5. The Further Education Staff College, Coombe Lodge, Blagdon, Bristol Reproduced by permission of the Further Education Staff College

Chapter 11
Skills of
Group Work

Summary

This chapter is about the skills of informal, participative group work. It begins by identifying the characteristics of group work, and the responsibilities of the leader and group members. Practical points about group work are discussed, followed by suggestions on how to get groups going, run discussions and deal with difficulties. The chapter includes an exercise on planning a group meeting.

Group work is useful for raising clients' awareness of health issues, helping them to explore their own values and attitudes and to make decisions. It also helps people who are trying to change their behaviour in some way, such as by losing weight, stopping smoking or helping each other to cope with problems.[1]

Time and practice are needed for the development of group work skills, and special training is recommended.[2] Audio or videotapes of group work sessions can be made and analysed as a useful learning exercise.[3]

What is Group Work?

Group work differs from traditional teaching in a number of key ways. The educational aims and the roles of the educator and the clients are fundamentally different, and are summarized below.[4]

Characteristics of Group Work and Traditional Teaching

Group work

1. The group members are active participants

2. The educator has the role of group leader, guiding group members through educational experiences, and helping ("facilitating") their learning

Traditional teaching

The group members are passive

The educator is a teacher who distributes knowledge

3. Educational aims are normally to raise awareness, facilitate attitude change and decision making, and foster mutual support	Educational aims are usually concerned with increasing knowledge
4. Group members participate in planning and choosing the content of courses	Group members have no say in the content of courses
5. Learning is through discovery and enquiry	Learning is through remembering facts and practical skills
6. The emphasis is on co-operation and sharing between members	There is no active encouragement to share; there may even be competition to see who knows the most
7. Learning can take place anywhere including people's homes	Normally only takes place in designated centres
8. Expressing new ideas is encouraged	Little emphasis on creative expression
9. The group is intrinsically motivated because learning is based on the group's interests and concerns	The group is extrinsically motivated because learning is based on the interests and concerns identified by the teacher

It is clear from this that the group leader and group members have particular responsibilities.

Responsibilities of the Leader

These are to:
— help group members to identify and clarify their interests and needs;
— help to develop a relaxed atmosphere in which members feel able to be open and trusting with each other;
— guide members through educational experiences, for example asking questions, providing material to trigger discussion, or organising "buzz" groups;
— offer all her expertise to the group members, making it clear that they are free to accept or reject the offer;
— accept all contributions from course members in a positive way, valuing them individually and collectively.

Responsibilities of a Group Member

These are to:
— participate in the choice of course content;
— choose whether, and how much, to participate;
— identify his own goals and concerns;
— decide which challenges and risks he is prepared to take. For example, how much

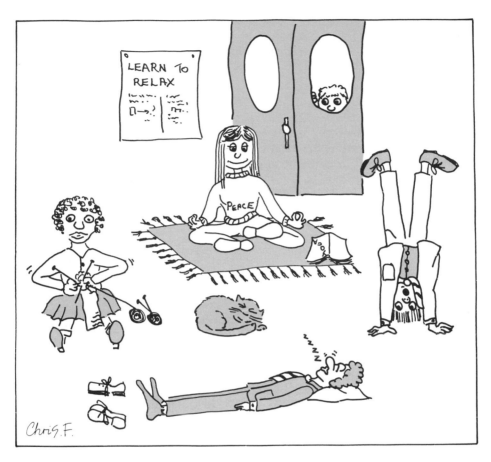

Group leaders can help to develop a relaxed atmosphere!

is he prepared to expose his own weaknesses and vulnerability to other people in the group?

It will probably be helpful to explain these responsibilities to a new group, particularly where members are accustomed to traditional teaching. For example, on meeting a new group, or a new member of a group, one might say "I'd like the time we spend together in this group to be as helpful to you as possible, so perhaps we might begin by discussing what *you'd* like to get out of these meetings. Then we can work out what topics we'll look at each week. I hope you'll all join in as much as possible, but no-one will be forced to." It may also be useful to remind people of the responsibilities of the leader and members at appropriate intervals, eg. "Let's remind ourselves about what we agree to do in the beginning . . .". "I suggest that there are several things we could do now—can we decide what will be most useful . . .?" "It's OK not to answer that question if you feel you'd rather not . . .".

Having established what group work is about, we now turn to the practicalities and skills involved.

Practical Points about Group Work

Practical points are concerned with numbers, time, location and seating.

Numbers

The ideal number of people in a group is usually considered to be between eight and twelve. If there are fewer than eight, people are likely to feel "exposed" and threatened; if more, it is difficult to get everyone involved, and shy members may find it hard to talk.

If large numbers are unavoidable, it may be more practical to form several small groups for specific tasks, such as sharing experiences.

Timing

Timing is crucial for the success of a group. Generally, the length of each session should be about 1½ hours, which gives enough time to break the ice and settle down to some useful work before concentration begins to flag. Short breaks or changes of activity help to keep the pace moving and to maintain interest. It is always best to end a group session when it is going well; never try to keep it going just for the sake of it if people are obviously tiring.

The day of the week and the time of day are also important. It is rarely possible to please everyone, and the constraints of the health professional's working day may leave little room for choice, but wherever possible, group members' views should be sought and taken into account.

Location

Location, too, can affect the success of a group. A hospital, clinic or health centre may appear clinical and cold to some people, and remind them of illness or pain. "Neutral" territory, such as a room in a pub or a community centre, or in someone's house, may be much more relaxing and inviting. If this is not possible, an unwelcoming room can be made to appear more friendly with easy chairs, cushions and background music.

Seating

Seating arrangements are an essential ingredient of successful participative group work. Seating people in a circle is best, with physical barriers to communication such as tables or desks removed. The circle symbolizes the equality of all members (including the leader), communication can flow across the group in any direction and all group members can see each other easily. It encourages members to talk to each other and not just to the leader (see Figure 5).

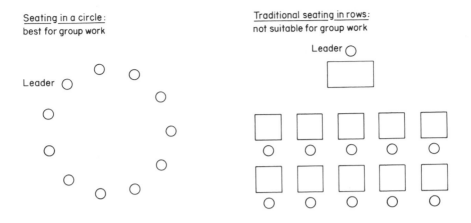

Figure 5. Seating for group work.

Getting Groups Going

Almost everyone feels nervous about going to a group meeting for the first time, especially if he is unlikely to know anyone there. The initial task for the group leader is to "break the ice" and help people to feel at ease.

On Arrival

It helps if clients can be greeted personally and introduced to other people—giving people something to do also helps: "Help yourself to a cup of tea!", "There are some books and leaflets on the table if you'd like to look at them till everyone has arrived".

Getting to Know Each Other

Knowing each person's name and something about him is the first step towards constructive groupwork because it helps him to feel valued as a member of the group, and is the beginning of openness and trust between members.

There are many ways of going about this, some of which are as follows:[5]

Introduction in pairs. Ask each person to sit next to someone he has not met before—one person in each pair then 'interviews' his partner. After a few minutes (the leader keeps the time) the partners swap roles and the other person is interviewed. Then, in turn, each member of the group introduces his partner by name and says something about him. You may like to remind people that no-one has to answer any questions if he does not wish to.

The leader could also suggest appropriate questions: in a parentcraft session, that partners find out if this is the first baby, where the mother goes for antenatal check-ups, or where she is booked to have her baby; in a slimming group, that people find out what diets their partners have tried.

Name games. Group members sit in a circle and you, the leader, take an object, such as a pen, and hand it to the person on your left, saying "My name is A and this is a pen". You ask the person who now holds the pen to say "My name is B and A says that this is a pen". B then passes the pen to the person on his left, who says "My name is C and B says that A says that this is a pen". This continues until the pen gets back to the beginning. If a group member forgets someone's name, the rest of the group can prompt him. This helps to establish a co-operative and supportive atmosphere as well as helping people to learn each other's names. Any tension and embarrassment are relieved by laughing and ice is effectively broken.

At subsequent group meetings, it is often helpful to do a quick round of names at the beginning, eg. "Who would like to have a shot at naming every member of the group?" or "I'm going to try to see if I can remember everyone's name".

You may like to set the tone by suggesting how people are addressed, by first names or more formally by Mr, Mrs etc. The important thing is to encourage people to use whatever feels comfortable. "My name is Ann Jones, and I'm happy for you to call me Ann if you like".

Sharing initial feelings and expectations. People may be helped to relax if they know that others also feel nervous or shy. So ask "What did you feel about coming here today? Did anyone feel nervous? Did anyone almost *not* come?"—this can open the way for people to express their anxieties. You can also encourage them to say why they have come to the meeting and what they expect to gain from it. It might help to ask members to complete a checklist, ticking statements that are true for them. Such statements could include:[6]

—I'm afraid I won't have anything to say
—I'm afraid I'll talk too much
—I'm worried I'll make a fool of myself
—I'll be too embarrassed to join in
—I'm afraid I might get upset
—I'm afraid I may be bored
—I want to meet other people in the same boat
—I enjoy talking to others
—I enjoy a good argument
—I want to get out of the house
—I want to go somewhere different
—I enjoy listening to other people

Each person can then compare his list with those of one or two other people in the group, and it may be helpful to share what has been discovered with the whole group.

Discussion Skills

It is a fallacy to believe that leading a discussion will just happen by putting a group of people together and saying "Let's discuss . . .". Discussion needs planning and preparation, and there are many ways of triggering it off and providing structures which help everyone to participate. Some of these are as follows.

Trigger Materials

Discussion can be triggered off by providing a focus, preferably a controversial one. This can simply be a question ("What do you think about the decision to close the cottage hospital?"), or it might be a leaflet, a poster, a short film, or something in a newspaper or magazine ("What do you think the makers of this cigarette are trying to convey in this advertisement?"). Choose something that people are likely to have strong views about.

Some health education films are specially made as trigger materials, presenting situations for people to talk about. Helpful notes for group leaders often accompany such films.

Brainstorms

This is a useful way to open up a subject and collect everyone's ideas. Ask an open question to which there is no single right answer ("Why do people drink?" "What do you feel you need to know before your baby is born?"). Accept every suggestion, without comment or criticism, and write them down in a list on a flipchart or blackboard. Ask the group not to start discussing the ideas until everybody has finished. You can make your own suggestions and write them down along with everyone else's.

In this way all members' contributions are equally valued, and everyone has a chance to participate. Encourage shy members by asking "Anything else?" and allowing silent pauses while people think.

Then you can set the group to work by asking them to put the ideas into categories, and to identify the key features of each category. For example, people might categorize reasons for drinking into a "constructive" category ("It helps me to socialize", "It helps me to relax, to feel good") and an "escape" category ("I can forget my problems", "It stops me from feeling upset").

Rounds

A "round" is a way of giving everyone an equal chance to participate. You invite each group member, in turn round the circle, to make a brief statement. You may like to start the round yourself or to join in when your turn comes in the circle. For example, ask everyone to make a brief statement about one of the following:

"My first feelings when I knew I was pregnant were . . ."
"What I think about jogging is . . ."
"The main reason why I can't lose weight is . . ."
"The thing which has helped me most is . . ."

There are three essential rules for successful rounds, which must be explained, and gently enforced if necessary. These are:
— no interruptions until each person has finished his statement;
— no comments on anybody's contribution until the full round is completed (ie. no discussion, praise, interpretation, criticism or I-think-that-too type of remark);
— anyone can choose not to participate. Give permission, clearly and emphatically,

that anyone who does not want to make a statement can just say "pass". This is very important for reinforcing the principle of voluntary participation.

Rounds are also useful ways of beginning and ending sessions. For example:

"One thing I've put into practice since last week is . . ."
"The main thing I've got from today's session is . . ."
"One thing I'm going to find out by next time we meet is . . ."

It's also a useful way of getting feedback. For example:

"One thing I really liked about today's session was . . ."
"One thing I didn't like about today's session was . . ."
"One thing I wish we'd done is . . ."

Buzz Groups

Buzz groups are small groups of two to six people who discuss questions or topics for short periods, usually about ten minutes. It is especially useful for large groups to be divided up in this way, as it gives everyone more chance to talk. Divide the groups first of all, and then say what you would like each one to do ("Make a list of the times when you want a cigarette" or "Talk about the things which you find helpful when you feel stressed"), and how long they have in which to do it. If you want people to share ideas with the rest of the group as a whole afterwards, it may be helpful to provide large sheets of paper and felt-tip pens, so that "posters" can be put up for everyone to see and discuss.

Safe Revelations

Sometimes people may hesitate or refuse to say what they really feel for fear of looking silly, being embarrassed or getting upset. One way of overcoming this is to give each person a piece of paper and ask him to write down (for example) what his biggest worry is, or what he really wants to know. All the papers are then folded and put in a receptacle such as a waste-paper basket or a shopping bag. Each person in turn picks out one piece of paper and reads aloud what it says. Tell people not to say if they happen to pick out their own piece of paper, and that, of course, nobody needs to identify himself as the author of any of the statements.

The aim is to find out the concerns of the group members in the security of anonymity. Make sure that everyone listens and does not comment until all the papers have been read out. Then you can discuss what was discovered.

Exercise — Planning a group meeting

1. Identify a health education opportunity that you have encountered or are likely to encounter, where informal group work would be appropriate.

continued on next page

continued

(For example, this could be a group of food handlers, a preretirement group, an antenatal group, a group of patients in hospital recovering from a heart attack, a stop-smoking group or a slimming group.)

Assume that your group consists of about 12 people who do not know each other, and that this is the first of several meetings.

2. What do you think would be the best place, time, and physical features of the meeting room?
3. What are your aims for the first meeting?
4. What are your objectives for your group members for the first meeting?

Complete the following:
"At the end of the first meeting, each group member will

1.   . . . . . .
2.   . . . . . .
3.   . . . . . .
etc   . . . . . .

5. Make a plan for what you will do
   — as people start to arrive
   — to get people to know each other
   — in the main part of the group meeting
   — to round off the meeting at the end
   — to evaluate whether you have achieved the objectives you set in (4) above).

Dealing with Difficulties

Health professionals often find the prospect of group work daunting, and anticipate being unable to cope with problems. A way forward is to acknowledge and face these fears, and work out strategies of coping should the problem actually arise. Some common fears and possible strategies for coping are as follows.

Silence

Are you afraid that you may be left with your group in an awful silence? If so, remember that silence can be useful; it can be time which group members need to think. Silence often does not feel as threatening to group members as it may do to you.

However, you may find it helpful to:
— run a group with a partner, so that you can help each other out if either of you gets stuck;
— ensure thorough preparation, so that you have planned activities and questions. Write down a plan, and a list of questions to ask (eg. at the end of a trigger film) and don't be afraid to refer to it in front of the group.
— have a "spare" activity ready to use if the cause of "drying up" is that what you have planned does not seem to be working.

Disasters

Unexpected "disasters" include such things as getting lost and arriving late, or finding that too few, or too many people have turned up. There is no blueprint strategy to cope with the unexpected, but it will help if you acknowledge what has happened and share it with your group ("I'm delighted that so many of you have come along, but I wasn't expecting such a crowd, so we may be a bit squashed this week"). Also share your plans for dealing with the "disaster" ("I'm going to try to get a bigger room next time" . . . "I'm going to start ten minutes late"). Sharing the problem and enlisting co-operation can have the positive benefit of encouraging mutual support; *not* sharing it can leave your group feeling angry.

Distractions

Distractions can take many forms: noises outside the room (eg. road works), noises inside the room (eg. crying babies, coughing), people coming in late or leaving early, interruptions. Distractions can also be caused by group members themselves, for example, by becoming very angry or upset.

As a rule, there are three choices for you as group leader:
—ignore them. This is seldom a good idea, as it leaves people wondering if you are going to do anything, and this in itself is a distraction.
—acknowledge and accept them. This is generally best with things you cannot change ("I know the traffic is really noisy, but there's nothing we can do about it, so I think we'll just have to put up with it").
—do something about them, preferably involving the group in the decision ("As so many of you found it difficult to get here by 2 pm, shall we start at 2.15 next week?" "Do you think it would be helpful if you took it in turns to look after the babies in the next room?").

If someone is showing emotion, such as crying, acknowledge it ("I can see that you're upset"), offer reassurance that it is OK to show emotion ("there's no need to be embarrassed . . . we don't mind if you cry . . ."), and offer the opportunity to talk about it ("Would you like to tell us what is upsetting you?") or to take some time away from the group, accompanied by you or someone else ("Shall we go outside for a few minutes?"). Do not put any pressure on the person; help him to do what he wants to do, whether it is talking, keeping silent, staying, leaving or being by himself. But do not ignore a show of emotion; ignoring it will only cause tension and embarrassment.

Difficult Behaviour

The way group members behave can pose difficulties for the leader. There are two broad categories of difficult behaviour: non-participation and talking too much. The latter category takes many forms, such as the know-all who always chips in with all the "answers", people who launch into long stories, people who interrupt, people who do not let other people get a word in edgeways, people who talk off the point, people who always disagree and people who always crack jokes.

A starting point for dealing with these difficulties is to try to think *why* people behave like this. Are they nervous, threatened, worried? Are they desperately in need of attention? If you can deal with the underlying cause, the situation is likely to improve. Secondly, note that people often change their behaviour as they get to know others and feel more comfortable in a group. Thirdly, try getting people to work in pairs or small groups, which can help quiet members to join in, and give others a break from the constant talker. Fourthly, use structures in your discussion such as "rounds" or make a point of asking for other people's opinions ("Would someone else like to say what he thinks?" "Would you like to give us your opinion, Ann?"). Finally, it may be necessary to confront the difficult person (not in front of the rest of the group!). For example, you could say: "I've noticed that you contribute a great deal to the group discussions. That makes me concerned about whether other people are getting enough chance to talk. I'd like to suggest that you keep your comments to just a couple of sentences. Would you feel OK about doing that?" (see the section *Giving feedback* in Chapter 10).

Notes, References and Further Reading

1 See Chapter 12, and the references in Chapter 12, for specific group work methods, on role-play, for example.

Other useful further reading on group work skills:

Rice B (1981) *Informal Methods in Health and Social Education.* Manchester: TACADE

(This book refers to school work, but much of it is also applicable to adult groups.)

Brown A (1979) *Group Work.* London: Heinemann Educational Books

(Although intended for social workers, this is a useful book for health educators.)

Stanton N (1982) *The Business of Communicating.* Harmondsworth: Pan Books

(Chapter 5 is about communicating in groups; it deals with broader issues such as group decision making, interaction patterns and leadership styles. Written for the business world, but useful for health educators.)

The Open University, Community Education (1983) *Group Notes*

(This booklet is written to help people running informal group discussions on parent and health issues, based on Open University Community Education material. It is a mine of clear, straightforward information and help for people new to running groups.) Obtainable from: Community Education, The Open University, Walton Hall, Milton Keynes, MK7 6AA

The *Group Notes* book is part of every pack of Community Education materials. There are Packs available on a number of different themes;
　　Looking After Yourself (health)
　　Women and Young Children
　　Parents Talking—the Developing Child
　　Racism in the Workplace and Community

2 *Working with Groups* is a Health Education Council/TACADE project designed to develop the group work skills of health professionals. Short courses are run by

health education officers and others in various parts of the country. There is a book and accompanying videotape designed to help people who teach group work skills, but useful for people who are learning as well. The book is available separately.

Satow A & Evans M (1983) *Working with Groups.* A TACADE/Health Education Council joint publication

Further details of the project from: TACADE, 2 Mount Street, Manchester M2 5NG

3   See: Perkins E R & Anderson D C (1981) *Self-assessment in the National Health Service.* Nafferton Books.

(Chapter 3 describes how group work can be tape-recorded and analysed.)

4   Based on ideas in:

Knowles M S (1972) *The Modern Practice of Adult Education . . . Andragogy versus Pedagogy.* New York: Association Press

5   There are many more "games" for teachers and group leaders, including "name games" and "ice-breakers", in:

Brandes D & Phillips H (1977) *Gamesters Handbook.* London: Hutchinson

Brandes D (1982) *Gamesters 2.* Leeds: Access Publishing

(Available from TACADE, 2 Mount Street, Manchester M2 5NG.)

6   Adapted, with kind permission, from:

The Open University, Community Education (1983) *Group Notes.* Open University, p 10

Chapter 12
Helping People
to Make
Health Choices

Summary

This chapter is about helping people to make health choices. The first section
looks at strategies for increasing self-awareness, clarifying values and
changing attitudes; the second section covers strategies for decision making
and the third deals with strategies for changing behaviour. The final section
discusses principles for using these strategies effectively. The chapter includes
an awareness-raising exercise and a case study on changing behaviour.

In this chapter we look at the skills and methods the health educator can use when
her aim is to help people to make choices about health and to carry them out.[1] Much
health behaviour appears to have developed without conscious decision-making; it
has "just happened" in response to individual or group circumstances and pressures.
Active decision-making is different because it involves commitment, time and energy
by both clients and the health educator.

Making health choices and carrying them out may bring benefits—these are not
only the benefits that go with a more health-promoting lifestyle, but also increased
self-esteem from the feeling of taking active control over a part of one's life, such
as being in control of the smoking habit rather than cigarettes being in control.[2]

However, it has to be accepted that people may prefer to carry on with "unhealthy"
behaviour, because, to them, it is not "unhealthy" as the benefits outweigh the risks.
The health educator should respect people's different points of view and their right to
choose. Furthermore, choosing a "healthy" behaviour does not automatically lead to
practising it. Changes such as taking more exercise, practising relaxation, going for
screening tests, wearing ear protectors in noisy surroundings, eating different foods and
stopping smoking are all hard work, and these changes in themselves may be stressful.
Social or economic circumstances may also prevent people from carrying out new
health behaviours, even if they would like to. Helping people to look at themselves,
their values and attitudes, and to make and carry out decisions which will result

in a healthier life, can be a most rewarding aspect of a health professional's work. We now turn to the strategies and skills she requires. (These strategies relate to four of the health education goals that were discussed in Chapter 2: self-awareness, attitude change, decision-making and behaviour change.)

Strategies for Increasing Self-awareness, Clarifying Values and Changing Attitudes

Traditional teaching operates in the hope that the "right" attitudes and values will be "caught" by learners. In contrast, we suggest that health education requires people to think critically about their values and build up their own value system. The process starts with raising self-awareness about health and continues through value clarification and growing commitment, until the value becomes a consistent aspect of the person's behaviour or character (see the "*Examples of health education goals*" in Chapter 2). This involves a change of attitude.[3]

Some strategies which are useful for increasing self-awareness, clarifying values and changing attitudes are described below—most of them are designed for group teaching, but some can be used with individuals.

Ranking or Categorizing

Ranking is a way of analyzing an issue in order to distinguish the relative importance of its different aspects. For example, in the exercise in Chapter 1 "*What does being healthy mean to you?*" readers are asked to rank aspects of "being healthy". This is a values clarification exercise, designed to help people to analyse "health" and decide which aspect of health is the most important to them.

Another approach is to generate a list of items, and then code them into different categories. The following exercise illustrates this approach; it is designed to raise awareness of the link between enjoyment and health.

Exercise — Enjoyment and health

Quickly list as many things as you can think of that you enjoy doing. Write them down the left-hand side of a piece of paper. On the right-hand side, code each item according to the following categories.

£   — any items that involve spending money
A   — any items that you do alone
P   — any items that you do with other people
R   — any items that involve some kind of risk
F   — any items that help to keep you fit
C   — any items that involve creativity
D   — any items that involve consumption of drugs (including alcohol and tobacco)
H +   — any items which positively affect your health
H −   — any items which negatively affect your health

continued on next page

---

continued

Items may be coded in more than one category. For example, if one of the things you enjoy doing is going out for a drink in a pub, this may be coded £, P and D.

What have you learnt about enjoyment and health through doing this exercise?

Using Polarized Views

This is a way of getting people to clarify their views about a particular issue. Views about the issue are polarized—that is, phrased to reflect extremely different views. For example, if the issue was "Is jogging good for you?" polarized views could be summed up as "Jogging kills people and only very fit athletes should do it" or "Jogging is very beneficial to health and all people would be fitter if they took it up". Examples of polarized views can be described by the group leader or taken from writings which express opposite views.

The group leader may ask people to work in pairs, with each individual acting as if he fully adopted one of the points of view for the duration of the exercise, whatever his personal opinions may be. First, each person writes down all the arguments he can think of which support his position, without discussing it with his partner at this stage. After a few minutes, the partners are asked to start arguing their case, usually for about 15 minutes. The leader then lists the points in favour of each view by asking each pair in turn to contribute one point, until all the points have been collected. She then asks the group to comment on what they have learnt. In this way, members of the group can consider a whole range of arguments, which helps them to understand other people's points of view, tolerate differences of opinion, clarify their own views, and perhaps see the issue in a new light.

Another example of a values clarification exercise using the polarized arguments approach is the exercise *Analysing your philosophy of health education* in Chapter 3, where readers are asked to consider arguments for and against two polarized views about the aim of health education.

Using a Values Continuum

This is an extension of the polarized argument technique. It helps people to understand the spread of opinion on a particular issue, and to clarify where they stand.

The leader describes two extremes of opinion and asks the group to imagine that these can be represented by two points, A and B, joined by a straight line. With a small group this line can be across a room; with a large group it could be drawn on the blackboard. The group members are then asked to mark or place themselves at a point along the line that best reflects their own view. For instance, in the jogging example discussed above, pro-joggers place themselves at one end, with the most extreme at the farthest point, people with moderate views stand around the middle, and the most ardent anti-jogger stands at the other end. The leader asks each person to state his views briefly as he takes up his position. Other people are asked not to interrupt or comment until everyone has taken up a position, or passed if they choose not to participate.

This technique can encourage a more detailed discussion of the range of possible options than the polarized argument technique. On the other hand, if everyone seems moderate, a better discussion may be stimulated by the polarized argument technique.

The values continuum technique is used in the last task of the exercise *Analysing your philosophy of health education* in Chapter 3.

Using Role Play

Role play generally means taking on the role of another person in a specified situation, and acting out what that other person might do and say in that situation. This helps people to understand what it feels like to be in another person's shoes. For example, adults role-playing an unemployed young person may be helped to understand feelings of rejection and boredom. Health professionals role-playing non-English-speaking patients visiting a clinic may be helped to understand how those patients feel, especially if the role-play is given added authenticity by using a foreign language which the health professionals do not speak.

It is also possible to role-play oneself in a new situation. This is a useful way of practising a new skill or rehearsing for a future event. For example, patients can role-play a consultation with a doctor in order to practise the skills of presenting their health problems to doctors.[4]

For an example of a role-play exercise, see *Skills of patient education* in Chapter 13.[5]

Playing Games

By "games" we mean structured activities, usually for a group of people, but sometimes for one or two people only. Games are a very useful teaching tool, because they can help to achieve a variety of aims. One is to help people to get to know each other ("ice-breakers"), such as the name games described in the section *Getting groups going* in Chapter 11. Other games can be devised which help people to trust each other, to communicate more openly or learn to relax.[6]

Other games in health education resemble traditional board or card games, and are designed to stimulate self-awareness and attitude change. For example, "White Monopoly" is an adaptation of the board game Monopoly, and aims to help people to examine their own racism.[7] "Workshuffle" is a set of cards which can be used to clarify values and attitudes towards work.[8]

Strategies for Decision-making

Making decisions—that is, choosing between alternative options—is a highly complex process, and a thorough exploration is outside the scope of this book.[9] However, it is useful to note that the basic process involves helping others to:
—define their situation or problem;
—identify their goals;
—generate alternative ways to reach those goals;
—weigh up the pros and cons of the alternatives;

—consider the likely consequences of pursuing each alternative;
—decide which is the best alternative.

Health professionals will often be involved in helping people who are faced with a choice, such as which treatment to have, whether to "do something" about a health problem or "let nature take its course", what to do about some other particular problem. Ultimately, the decision is the client's but the health educator can help by guiding the client through the stages of decision making, asking key questions and giving relevant information ("If you do X what's likely to happen is . . .", "If you do Y the chances are that . . .", "You might find it helpful to consider that . . ." and so on).

If, for example, a health professional has the task of helping a patient to decide what to do about having her baby vaccinated, the stages could be to:
—*define the problem.* For example, is the parent worried about having the child vaccinated at all, or is it just the whooping cough vaccination which is worrying? Is it *when* to have the child vaccinated, or *if?*
—*identify the goal:* the child to have the best possible chance of staying healthy.
—*define the alternatives:* no vaccinations at all, some vaccinations, or all vaccinations?
—*weigh up the pros and cons:* what is the available information on the risks from catching the disease compared with the risks of having the vaccination?
—*consider the likely consequences of pursuing each alternative:* for the child, in terms of health risk; for the parent, in terms of anxiety, guilt and responsibility;
—*decide which is the best course of action.*

Strategies for Changing Behaviour

Having made a choice, based on their own values, people may need considerable help to carry their decision through into action. A number of techniques developed from behavioural psychology are useful, and the philosophy behind them (that people are responsible for their own behaviour and are capable of exercising control over it) is as important as the techniques themselves.[10] A variety of materials has been developed to help people to change different aspects of their behaviour, such as stopping smoking, controlling drinking, changing eating habits and taking up exercise.[11] Some useful techniques are as follows.

Self-monitoring

Self-monitoring is keeping a detailed and precise account, often in the form of a diary, of behaviour which is to be changed. Its aim is to help people to analyse their pattern of behaviour and become fully aware of what they are doing, which is a starting point for gaining control. Secondly, the "diary" provides a base-line against which progress can be checked.

Self monitoring involves answering questions such as:
—how frequently does the problem occur?
—when the problem occurs, what else is happening both externally (in the environment), and internally (in thoughts and feelings)?

—what event leads up to the problem?
—what happens afterwards: the consequences?

An example of a Smoker's Diary is given below.

Example of self-monitoring — a smoker's diary

Day . . . . (Complete one of these charts every day)

Each time you smoke a cigarette, note down in the columns:

1   the time
2   how urgent your craving for a cigarette is, on a scale of 1–10
    (1 = very little craving, 10 = extremely high craving)
3   where you smoke the cigarette
4   whether you are alone or who you are with
5   do you smoke it with drinks (coffee, tea, alcohol)
6   do you smoke it after a meal
7   what else are you doing at the time (eg. chatting, reading the paper,
    working, talking on the phone)
8   why did you decide to smoke this cigarette
9   what do you feel about it afterwards

Time	Craving	Where	Who with	With drinks	After meal	Doing what	Why	Afterwards

Total number of cigarettes smoked today = _____

Identifying Costs, Benefits and Rewards

The cost of changing behaviour can be considerable, involving deprivation of "crutches", such as cigarettes, and pleasures, such as eating and drinking, or there may be a heavy price to pay in terms of time, effort and perhaps money. So it is helpful to identify the benefits clearly, and set up a system of rewards to encourage perseverance.

Benefits may be long-term, such as better health or increased life-expectancy. They may be abstract ("It will prove I've got will-power") or in other people's interests ("for the family's sake"). Important though these benefits may be, it is also necessary to find immediate, short-term rewards which people genuinely enjoy, such as small treats.[12]

Setting Targets and Evaluating Progress

Targets should be realistic rather than idealistic. Losing an average of one pound in weight a week is realistic for most people; losing a stone in a month usually is not. People may have unrealistic hopes and expectations about what can be achieved, which leads to disappointment and a sense of failure when the target has not been met.

In order to evaluate progress, it is necessary to keep a record of behaviour so that achievements can be seen clearly. Progress should be assessed once the "new" behaviour has been given a fair trial perhaps for two or three weeks, although short-term reviews ("How have I done today?") can also be useful.

If the target is not being achieved, possible reasons must be looking for and changes made. For example:
— is the target too difficult? Should it be lowered?
— are the rewards too distant? Is there a more immediate reward which could be more encouraging?
— is there an unforseen crisis or illness? If so, encouragement to continue self-monitoring and look on the setback as a learning experience may be needed.
— are other people unhelpful? More strategies to cope with the negative influence of other people may be needed.
— are there other problems which require help, such as learning to cope with anxiety or stress?

Devising Coping Strategies

Changing behaviour can mean coping with numerous difficulties, for at least a short period of time, until the new behaviour becomes a normal part of life. Someone who is stopping smoking has to cope with problems such as the craving he feels, the need to put something in his mouth, not knowing what to do with his hands, doing without his accustomed "tension-reliever" in moments of stress, and resisting the offer of a cigarette.

People adopt a wide variety of coping strategies, and it is often useful to get a group to share their ideas about what helps them to cope.[13] The list of strategies here is certainly not exhaustive.
— finding a substitute, such a substituting chewing gum or herbal cigarettes for the real thing, or eating low-calorie foods instead of high-calorie ones;
— changing some routines and habits which are closely associated with the "problem" behaviour. Examples are drinking tea or fruit juice instead of coffee, because coffee is closely associated with cigarettes;
— making it difficult to carry on with the "problem" behaviour, by, for example, keeping cigarettes in an inconvenient place, sitting in a no-smoking compartment, and deciding to restrict eating to mealtimes, not between meals.

What all these strategies have in common is that they require only a small step to achieve a large degree of help for self-control. Other strategies may be:
— getting support from other people "in the same boat", who might be from a slimming group, an anti-smoking clinic, or a self-help group. Another helpful way of getting support is by linking with another person on the understanding that

each may telephone or meet the other if either of them needs help[14] (see Chapter 14 for further reading on self-help groups).

— practising ways of responding to unhelpful social pressures, for example, refusing the offer of a cigarette or a drink.

— adopting a one-day-at-a-time approach. The prospect of the whole of the rest of life without a cigarette may be overwhelming, but the prospect of one day without one is far more tolerable. Even shorter time-spans may be helpful, such as putting off eating, drinking or smoking for just five minutes at a time.

— learning relaxation techniques and other ways (such as exercise) of relieving stress. Simple relaxation routines which can be practised at any time and place can be helpful in coping with stressful moments when the "old" reaction would have been to reach for a drink or a cigarette.

Case study — Changing behaviour in practice

Joan is divorced. She has a toddler who constantly wakes her at night. She has used various stratagems, including trying to tire him out physically just before bedtime, keeping him up later, leaving toys for him to play with in the night, and playing with him herself in the night. She has started to have a few glasses of sherry in the evenings to help her to relax and now finds that she needs another sherry to help her get back to sleep after getting up in the night.

She goes to her doctor for help. He explains that the stratagems she used to try to get her son to sleep do not work because they merely stimulate him and give him rewards (playing and getting attention from his mother) when he wakes up. He suggests that the toddler needs to learn to relax before he goes to bed. The doctor asks Joan if she knows anything which seems to help her child to relax, and using her suggestions they devise a suitable bedtime routine for Joan to try out.

Turning to Joan herself, the doctor asks how she has been coping and Joan responds that a few sherries in the evening helped at first but now she is worried that she may be relying too much on drinking to help her to cope. He then asks about her reasons for drinking. She has already identified that it helps her to cope; it makes her feel less anxious and "strung up". She says "When I've had a hard day I deserve a drink . . . it helps me relax and forget my problems for a while".

The doctor asks her to think of reasons why drink may not be the most helpful way to reward herself, help herself to relax or solve her problems. He suggests that she should think about alternatives, such as leisure activities. He tells her about a local mother-and-toddler group where she can meet other mothers in similar circumstances. He suggests that she keeps a drinker's diary so that they can together find out more about her drinking patterns and help her to set limits on her drinking. He shows her an example of a drinker's diary and explains how to count each drink using standard measures. Joan agrees to fill it in every time she has a drink during the next fortnight.

Finally, he asks Joan to come back and see him in two weeks' time to discuss whether the new routines are helping the toddler to sleep and to see

continued on next page

continued

what she has discovered from the suggestions he has made. He also arranges for the health visitor to visit Joan in a few days time.

What strategies does the doctor use to help Joan with her problems? What other strategies could he have used?

Using Strategies Effectively

We have discussed a number of different strategies which health educators can use when they are trying to help clients to increase their self-awareness, clarify their values, change attitudes and change behaviour. In order to use these strategies with maximum effect, there are a number of principles to bear in mind.

Making Healthier Choices Easy Choices

People do not make health choices in a vacuum; they make them in the context of their own environment, subject to all the pressures and influences that surround them. If this environment is conducive to a healthier lifestyle, clients have greater freedom to choose the "healthier" alternatives and change their behaviour. For example, the provision of cycleways makes it easier to take regular exercise by cycling to work; provision of litter bins, combined with frequent emptying, helps people to Keep Britain Tidy; a no-smoking policy in public places such as restaurants and cinemas helps people not to smoke. National and local policies can create a climate where it is easier to adopt healthier behaviour. (See the section *What affects health?* in Chapter 1.)

Relating to Clients

Research consistently shows that the degree of client change is related to helper empathy; in other words, clients are more likely to change if the health educator understands the client, sees things from his point of view, and accepts him on his own terms (this has been discussed at more length in Chapter 8 *Relationships with Clients*). Achieving this relationship may be the most difficult part of helping people to change.[15] Furthermore, the attitude and behaviour of the health educator herself is likely to influence the outcome. For example, doctors who themselves smoke are less likely to be effective in helping people to choose to stop smoking.[16]

Using Learning Methods Sensitively

People invest a great deal of emotion in their values and attitudes, which means that the exercises we have described here, especially those that are designed to encourage people to explore feelings, such as role-play, need to be handled with care and sensitivity. Special training in the use of experiential teaching methods is recommended, but at the very least, group leaders should not attempt to use them unless they have experienced them first themselves. Some points to remember are as follows.

—Explain the activities carefully and thoroughly, and check to ensure that everybody understands what the exercise is for, and what they are expected to do.

—Emphasize that participation is entirely voluntary.

—Allow plenty of time for discussion at the end. If people's opinions and cherished ideas have been challenged, they are likely to feel strongly about it. Increased self-awareness may be a very uncomfortable experience, too. The group leader should ensure that people have time to express their feelings and get any support that they need before they leave the group.

—Ensure that there is an atmosphere of confidentiality and trust, so that people feel free to explore their views and feelings in safety. If they feel they may be laughed at or gossiped about, they will not participate fully, if at all.

—Save your own views to the end, after the group members have had a chance to think things through for themselves. Be open and honest about yourself and your values, and if you, too, are confused, say so!

Using Emotional Appeals

The "shock-horror" approach to health education was much used in the 60s and 70s, when cancerous lungs and the wasted bodies of drug addicts were depicted in order to scare people away from cigarettes and drugs. But this approach has now been shown to have little to recommend it. It can be counter-productive because people think "It will never happen to me" and dismiss such horrors from their minds. It can induce guilt and anxiety in people who feel unable to change, and can be harmful to those who are already anxious and vulnerable.

At best, the shock-horror approach may produce a short-term attitude change, or perhaps act as trigger to action which would probably have happened anyway. If this approach *is* used, it should be accompanied by a clear message about what to do to avoid the depicted dangers, and provision needs to be made for long-term support in carrying out the recommended actions.

Taking a Long-term View

Changes in attitude and behaviour may take a long time, and single sessions by health educators are unlikely to have much effect, unless they are part of a long-term strategy. Follow-up work is very important. For example, evaluation of the Give Up Smoking (GUS) kits designed to assist general practitioners to help patients to stop smoking, suggests that those GPs who make follow-up appointments are more likely to be effective.[17]

Notes, References and Further Reading

1 For further reading on the theory of attitude and behaviour change, see:

Kanfer F H & Goldstein A P (1980) *Helping People Change—a Textbook of Methods*. Oxford: Pergamon Press

An Open University Community Education Course *Health Choices* aims to help people to understand their own health, how much control they have over it and the choices they can make. Further details from: The Open University, PO Box 76, Milton Keynes MK7 6AN. The book which forms the core of the course is available separately:

Open University (1980). *The Good Health Guide*. Harmondsworth: Pan Books (originally published by Harper and Row)

2 For an example see:

Langer E J & Rodin J (1976) The effects of choice and enhanced social responsibility: a field experiment in an institutional setting. *J Pers Soc Psychol*, 34, 191–198

(This study showed that residents in a home for the elderly who were given personal responsibility and choice showed improved alertness, active participation and self-rated well being when compared with control subjects.)

3 See:

Keeton M T *et al* (1976) *Experiential Learning*. London: Josey-Bass

Simon S B *et al* (1972) *Values Clarification—a Handbook of Practical Strategies for Teachers and Students*. New York: Hart

Read D A *et al* (1977) *Health Education—the Search for Values*. Englewood Cliffs, NJ: Prentice-Hall

4 See:

Evans M, Rice W & Grey G (1981) *Free to Choose—an Approach to Drug Education*. Manchester: TACADE, Section 7—A Visit to the Doctor

5 For further reading on role-play see:

Van Ments M (1983) *The Effective Use of Role Play—a Handbook for Teachers and Trainers*. London: Kogan Page

Rice W (1981) Discussion, role-play and simulation in the classroom. In Cowley J, David K & Williams T (eds) *Health Education in Schools*. London: Harper and Row, Ch 13

6 For books of "games" see:

Brandes D & Phillips H (1977) *Gamesters Handbook*. London: Hutchinson.

Brandes D (1982) *Gamesters 2*. Leeds: Access Publishing (available from TACADE, 2 Mount Street, Manchester M2 5NG).

7 *White Monopoly* is available from: The National Youth Bureau, 17–23 Albion Street, Leicester LE1 6GD

8 *Workshuffle* is available from: Lifeskills Associates, "Ashling", Back Church Lane, Leeds LS16 8DN

9 For further reading on the sociopsychological factors involved in decisions and actions about health, see:

Becker M H *et al* (1977) Selected psychosocial models and correlates of individual health-related behaviours. *Medical Care*, 15 (5) supplement. (This is an account of the much-quoted Health Belief Model.)

Tones B K (1979) Past achievement and future success. In Sutherland I (ed) *Health Education—Perspectives and Choices*. London: George Allen & Unwin, Ch 12

10 For a general textbook on self-control see:

Thoresen C E & Mahoney M J (1974) *Behavioural Self-Control.* New York: Holt,
Rinehart & Winston

11 East J R & Travers B A (1979) *No Smoke—a Psychologically-based Manual of
Information and Self-applied Exercises for Use in Giving up Smoking.* Kingston
Polytechnic, Kingston-upon-Thames, Surrey

Ruzek J (1982) *Drinkwatchers Handbook—a Guide to Healthy Enjoyment of Alcohol
and Methods to Achieve Sensible Drinking Skills.* Accept Publications, Western
Hospital, Seagrove Road, London SW6 1RZ

Health Education Council *That's The Limit* (booklet on drinking). London: Health
Education Council. An "eating diary" and an "exercise dairy" are included in
Look After Yourself, Community Education Study Package. Open University,
Walton Hall, Milton Keynes MK7 6AA

Simnett K I, Wright L & Evans M (1983) *Drinking Choices—a Training Manual
for Alcohol Educators.* London: Health Education Council/TACADE

12 Self-rewarding ideas are included in "Changing Your Ways?" in the *Look After
Yourself, Community Education Study Package.* Open University, Walton Hall,
Milton Keynes MK7 6AA

13 Many coping strategies are listed in leaflets from the Health Education Council
and the Scottish Health Education Group which deal with stopping smoking and
sensible drinking. See also a booklet produced by the West Midlands Health
Services *The People Say How They Gave Up Smoking,* available from Public
Relations Division, West Midland Regional Health Authority, Arthur Thomson
House, 146 Hagley Road, Birmingham B16 9PA.

14 For example, pairs who contact each other between group meetings are more likely
to be successful at ceasing to smoke than pairs who do not.

Janis I L *et al* (1970) Facilitating effects of daily contact between partners who
make a decision to cut down on smoking. *J Pers Soc Psychol,* **17**, 25–35

15 See, for example:

Carkhuff R F (1969) *Helping and Human Relations.* New York: Holt, Rinehart
Winston

Tuckett D (1983) *Final Report of the Patient Project.* London: Health Education
Council (on doctor-patient relationships)

16 Pincherle G *et al* (1970) Smoking habits of business executives: doctor variations in
reducing consumption. *Practitioner,* **205**, 209–212

17 Health Education Council *Give Up Smoking* kits for general practitioners

Chapter 13
Teaching
and
Instructing

Summary

The first section of this chapter uses an exercise to analyse the qualities
and abilities of a good teacher, then outlines some principles of effective
teaching. Subsequent sections contain guidelines on giving talks, strategies for
patient education and teaching practical skills. A role-play exercise on skills of
patient education is included.

This chapter is about the skills and methods of traditional teaching, when the health
education goals are primarily concerned with helping clients to acquire knowledge
or skills. Examples are giving a talk on a health topic to a large community group,
giving information to a patient about his diagnosis, treatment and self-care, teaching
a small group of clients techniques of relaxation, or instructing a patient how to test
his own urine samples for sugar.

We have focused on selected aspects of teaching which we identify as specially
relevant for health professionals. This chapter is certainly not comprehensive, and
further reading is recommended[1]; it should also be studied alongside others which
contain relevant material, especially Chapters 7, 8, 9, 10 and 16.

Health professionals generally have credibility because of their training and expert
knowledge. This is likely to be valued and respected by clients, but expertise alone
does not make a good teacher. The next section is concerned with identifying the
qualities and skills of a good teacher.

What Makes a Good Teacher?

Every health professional has spent many hours on the receiving end of other people's
teaching, and this in itself is a useful learning experience. The following exercise
will help health educators to identify factors which have helped and hindered their
own learning, and to assess their own qualities and abilities.

Exercise — What helps and hinders learning?

Think of two occasions when you have been a learner, such as when you were a student in class, or in the audience listening to a talk, or when you were being taught on a one-to-one basis. These occasions need not have been connected with work (for example, listening to an art lecture or taking a driving lesson). One should be when you felt, overall, that the teaching session was *good* and the other when it was *bad*. The aim of the exercise is to identify the factors that made them good or bad for you.

In each of your two situations in turn, identify factors which helped you to learn, and factors which hindered your learning. Think of these factors in three categories:

— factors to do with *the environment* (eg. too hot? noisy? hard chairs? a spacious, comfortable room?)
— factors to do with *the qualities of the teacher herself* (eg. sense of humour? appeared bored? contagious enthusiasm? seemed unfriendly?)
— factors to do with *the presentation* (eg. talked too long? used relevant illustrations? involved audience? muddled? used words you didn't understand? used audiovisual aids effectively?)

Enter these factors in on a chart:

	Environment	Teacher	Presentation
Factors which helped			
Factors which hindered			

If you are working in a group, compare your chart with those of other people.
What have you learnt about the importance of the environment?
What qualities of a good teacher do you think you already possess?
What helpful points about presentation do you think you already use in your own teaching?
What points about your own qualities or presentation would you like to improve?

We do not suggest that health professionals set out to change their personalities. The aim of identifying strengths and weaknesses is to provide a basis for developing skills.

Some Principles of Effective Teaching

Here we identify some basic principles which should be borne in mind in all teaching, whether to individuals or groups.

Work from the Known to the Unknown

Your starting point is what people know already; this is obvious common sense, but frequently overlooked. The result is that time is wasted by teaching people what they already know, or by talking over their heads. You need to find out as much as possible about what your clients already know. If you cannot do this in advance, spend some time at the beginning of the session asking a few questions. If you have a mixed audience with varying degrees of knowledge, it may be best to acknowledge that some people know more than others, and you will have to make a decision about the level at which to pitch your information: "Some of you will probably know this, but I'll talk about it briefly because it will be new to others . . .".

Your aim is build new information, or new skills, on to what is already known.

Aim for Maximum Involvement

People learn best if they are actively involved in the learning process, not just passively listening.

Firstly, try to involve your clients in deciding the aim and content of the teaching. If you are running a course, such as a series of antenatal classes or one on food hygiene, you might begin by explaining your aims, asking for comments and suggestions, and then going on to discuss the content. This will help to increase motivation by including clients' own interests and, hopefully, stimulating them to think about new areas. It also helps clients to recognize that they are responsible for their own learning. The goals and content of one-to-one teaching can always be established by mutual agreement at the beginning of a session.

As a general rule, it is worth considering how much room for negotiation there is in your teaching, and spending time to find out what people really want. Ask yourself: "Is what I teach what *I want to teach* or what *my clients want to learn?*"

Secondly, keep your clients involved as much as possible during teaching sessions. This is a challenge if you are giving a talk or a lecture to a large audience, but there are possibilities, such as asking people to respond to a question, eg. "I'd like you to put your hand up if you made a New Year resolution to take more exercise this year". Or ask them to respond to a series of statements: for example, as an introduction to a talk on nutrition, ask the audience to stand up, then ask them to sit down if they: usually eat white bread . . . add sugar to tea and coffee . . . regularly eat fried food . . . add salt at the table . . . . Most of them will be sitting down by now but they will feel alert and involved. Another way of keeping an audience involved is to give them time to talk. This can be done by having question-and-answer sessions, or by allowing short breaks when they can talk about something in groups of two or three for a few minutes. In a talk on passive smoking, for example, you could give your audience a couple of minutes to tell their neighbours how they find they are affected by other people's smoke.

You can also keep people involved with eye contact. Look members of your audience in the eye, and make sure that you look round at everybody, not just the people immediately in front of you.

Vary your Teaching Methods

It is natural to consider teaching from the teacher's point of view but it may be more helpful to look at it from the client's point of view. For example, talking for half an hour demands concentrated effort and total involvement on your part; but all your audience is doing is listening, which only involves one of their senses and is highly unlikely to hold their full attention for that length of time.

Bringing variety into health teaching can be done in many ways—these include strategies that can be used with individuals, groups, large audiences, children or adults.

Client involvement	*Materials and methods*
Listen	Lectures, audiotapes.
Read	Books, booklets, leaflets, handouts, posters, black/white board, flipchart, overhead projector transparency
Look	Photographs, drawings, paintings, posters, charts, material from magazines (such as advertisements), flannelgraphs
Look and listen	Films, videocassettes, tapeslide sets, slides with commentary, demonstrations
Listen and talk	Question-and-answer sessions, discussions, informal conversations, debates, brainstorming
Read, listen and talk	Case studies, discussions based on study questions or handouts
Read, listen, talk and actively participate	Drama, role-play, games, simulations, quizzes, practising skills
Read and actively participate	Programmed learning, computer-assisted learning
Make and use	Models, charts, drawings
Use	Equipment
Action research	Gathering information, opinions, interviews and surveys
Projects	Making health education materials—videos, leaflets etc
Visits	To health service premises, fire station, sewage works, play groups, voluntary organisations
Write	Articles, letters to the press, stories, poems

(For discussion of some of these methods, see Chapters 11 and 12; for discussion on the use of audiovisual aids, see Chapter 16.)

Ensure Relevance

When teaching you should ensure that, as far as possible, what you say is relevant to the needs, interests, and circumstances of the clients. For example, recommendations about health-promoting activities which cost money may be helpful to a relatively well-off audience, but not of much use to an audience which has no money for "extras". A discussion on vaccination may be irrelevant to a pregnant woman whose overwhelming concern is the birth itself; she may not relate to an issue which will not affect her until afterwards.

You will help your clients to see the relevance of your subject if you use concrete examples, practical problems and case studies to explain and illustrate your points. Abstract generalizations and quotations of huge figures are difficult to relate to. For example say "one person in ten" instead of "X million people in this country", tell the story of a home accident rather than describe a list of risk factors, and describe "increasing the risk" by saying "It's like driving a car with faulty brakes—there's

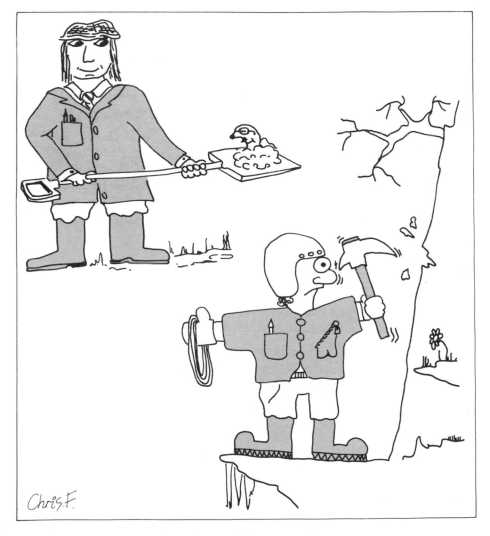

A common mistake is attempting too much . . . a well-moved molehill is better than an abortive attempt to shift Everest!

no guarantee that you will have an accident, but your chances of having one are greater".

Identify Realistic Goals and Objectives

We have already discussed (in Chapter 2) the importance of clearly identifying health education goals and educational objectives but it is worth emphasizing again how essential it is to be clear about what you are trying to do (raise awareness of a health issue? give people more health knowledge?) and what you want your clients to know, feel and/or do at the end of your teaching session. As we mentioned above, your clients may be involved in these decisions.

A common mistake is to attempt too much and talk for too long. Three or four key points is all that you can ever expect people to remember from a teaching session. Teaching more than that does not mean that they learn more; it usually means that they forget more. For example, if you are asked to give a talk on a huge theme, such as Food for Health, Avoiding Accidents, First Aid or Pollution, you will need to select what you feel to be the few points most relevant for your audience, and avoid the temptation to give an everything-you-ever-wanted-to-know-about talk. A well-moved molehill is better than an abortive attempt to shift Everest.

Organize your Material

Whether you are talking to a group or teaching an individual, it helps if you organize your material into a logical framework, and tell your client(s) what this is, both at the beginning, and during, your teaching session.[2]

For example, with an individual patient, say:
"I am going to tell you:
—what we have found to be wrong with you;
—the treatment I am going to suggest for you;
—how much time you will need off work.
Firstly, what we have found out is that . . .
Secondly, I think that the best treatment for you is . . .
Finally, about taking time off work, I think that you will probably need . . ."

The same principle applies if you are talking to a group. The old adage is: "Tell'em what you're going to tell 'em; tell 'em; then tell 'em what you've told 'em". This is sound advice, because it helps both you and the audience to know where you are and where you are going. "Flagging" where you are at intervals is helpful: "That's all I've got to say on the benefits of yoga; now, to move on to how you can get started . . .", or "Now I'd like to move on to my third and final point, which you may remember I said was about . . .".

Evaluation and Feedback

It is important to get feedback on your teaching, so that you can assess how much your client is learning and improve your own performance in the future (see sections *Stage 7: Plan evaluation methods* and *Stage 9: Evaluate* in Chapter 7, and the section *Asking questions and getting feedback* in Chapter 10).

Guidelines for Giving Talks

Giving a talk, or perhaps a formal lecture, is a frequent feature of a health educator's work. There are considerable disadvantages in this method: a talk is largely a one-way communication process with little opportunity to assess how much people are learning or understanding, and with only a small proportion of it likely to be remembered at the end and still less a few days later.

Despite these limitations, talks and lectures can be valuable for several reasons. A talk can be used to introduce a subject by giving a bird's-eye view of it, and this may lead people to take further action. For example, an introductory talk on first aid may lead people to enrol for a first-aid course. A talk may awaken a critical attitude in the audience, for example, by drawing their attention to issues such as lead pollution or the lack of understandable information on food labels. Many people do not read books and articles or habitually watch documentary programmes on television; for them, a talk may be an important source of health information. Giving talks is also a relatively economical way to use a health professional's time, since large numbers of people can be addressed at one time.

In addition to the general principles discussed in the last section there now follow some specific points which may help you to plan, and deliver, a successful talk.[3]

Check the Facilities

If possible, visit the place where you are going to give your talk, and check the seating, lighting and audiovisual equipment including electric power points and extension leads. On the day of the talk, arrive in good time so that you can arrange chairs, open windows, put up blackout and check that the equipment is working. Get your overhead projector, slide or film projector focused ready for use, and if you need blackout, check that you can turn the lights on and off quickly so that you do not lose rapport with the audience while they are left in the dark.

Making and Using Notes

It is generally best to give a talk from notes written on paper or cards. The more experienced you are the fewer notes you are likely to need, unless your talk is full of technical detail or likely to be taken down and quoted verbatim (eg. by the press). However, very few people can give a successful talk with no notes at all, and beginners may find it helpful to write out a talk in full before they transfer the main points to notes.

If you are writing out your talk in full to begin with, it is useful to know that a 50 minute lecture consists of about 5,000 words, allowing for pauses and an estimated speed of delivery of about 110 words per minute. You can then try transferring the key points as notes to cards or paper.

Never give a talk by writing it out in full and then reading it. Unless you are an exceptional orator who can "act" the lines, it will sound flat and stilted. Furthermore, you will find difficulty in looking at your audience, because you will need to keep your eyes on your notes, and once you look up you are likely to lose your place.

Prepare your Introduction

Secure the attention of audience with your opening words. Some ways of doing this are:
—state a startling fact;
—ask a question which has no easy answer;
—use a visual image to trigger interest;
—get the audience to do something active (some suggestions are discussed in the earlier section on *Aiming for maximum involvement*);
—tell a joke, if you have the confidence to do it successfully.

Establish eye contact with your audience and, if necessary, ask them if they can see and hear you.

State your aim and theme at the beginning of your talk ("Tell 'em what you're going to tell 'em"). It should be a brief statement, not a complex summary of the whole talk. For example, say "I'm going to talk about what to do if someone is unconscious, not breathing, bleeding or in a state of shock" but do not go into detail at this point about what the correct actions should be; save that for the main part of the talk.

By the time you have finished the introduction, you should have:
—established your aim and theme with the audience;
—obtained their interest and commitment;
—ensured that they can hear and see you clearly.

Prepare the Key Points

Identify the three or four main points you wish to make, and prepare your talk around each point in turn. Illustrate and support your points with evidence from your experience or from research, with examples, audiovisual materials, and so on. (See Chapter 16 on using and producing audiovisual materials, including leaflets, handouts, films and slides.)

Plan a Conclusion

You need to plan how you will end your talk in order to avoid rambling on or trailing off. Some ways of ending are:
—a very brief recapitulation (not a boring repetition) of what you've said—"We've now covered the basics of life-saving first aid".
—a statement of what you hope the audience will do with the information you have given them—"I hope that you can confidently do the right thing next time you have to help someone who's had an accident".
—a suggestion for further action—"If you'd like to learn more please come to see me afterwards".
—a question—"Don't you think that basic first aid is so simple and so important that it should be taught to every child in school?".
—thank the audience for their attention and/or participation.

Ask for Questions

If possible, include a question-and-answer session in your talk. It gives you feedback, and gives the audience a chance to participate.

When you ask for questions, allow people time to think; do not assume that there are to be no questions just because one is not instantly forthcoming. When a question is asked, it is often helpful to repeat or summarize it. This gives you a little time to consider the question, and ensures that everyone else in the audience has heard it. Never ignore or refuse to answer a question—if you don't know the answer say so, and ask anyone else in the audience if he does. In any case, this helps to involve the audience; you could also ask for comments on answers "Does anyone else have suggestions which could help the lady who asked that question?"

Work on your Presentation

Important points about presentation include pace and timing, which usually means having consciously to slow down your rate of speaking; the nervous beginner finds the silence of pauses to be threatening and wants to get the whole thing over! Other factors are looking at the audience and using notes appropriately.

Thorough preparation will help you to feel confident, but however nervous or inexperienced you may feel, do not apologize for being there. For example, if you have been asked to give a talk about your work, *do not* say "I'm going to talk about the work of health visitors, but I'm afraid I've only been qualified for a year so there's a lot I don't know yet". Instead, present yourself positively "I'm going to talk about the work of health visitors. I've been qualified for a year now, and I'd like to share my experience of the work with you".

The way to improve presentation is by practice. Practise giving your talk out loud, or to friends or colleagues. Ask a trusted colleague to sit in when you give a talk, and to give you feedback afterwards. It is even more helpful to see yourself on videotape, so that you can assess your own strengths and weaknesses.

Plan for Contingencies

A major fear when giving a talk is that you may "dry up" or lose your place. If this is a possibility, it is better to face it and think beforehand about what you will do if it should happen. It is best to acknowledge that you have a problem rather than leave an embarrassed silence. For example, say "Sorry, my mind seems to have gone blank" or "I've lost my place". Then remember that an audience is likely to be friendly rather than hostile and will probably want to help you. So let them help by asking for time: "Would you mind if I took a minute to get myself together" or "Excuse me for a moment while I look through my notes".

Another fear is that audiovisual equipment will break down. You cannot insure against this, so it is best to have a contingency plan ready. For example, "As we can't see the sequence on the film as I'd hoped, I'll write the stages up on the blackboard and talk through them instead" (see also the section *Dealing with difficulties* in Chapter 11).

Strategies for Patient Education

Research reports have shown that patients want information but have difficulty in understanding and remembering it.[4] Furthermore, in a summary of 68 studies which examined compliance with treatment regimes, dietary instructions and ante-natal advice, it was calculated that between 38 and 55 per cent of patients did not comply.[5] Another summary of research studies shows that only half of the patients on long-term treatment schedules actually follow the schedules prescribed.[6]

There are many reasons for these apparent failures, but it seems reasonable to suppose that some of the responsibility lies with the manner in which people give information, instructions and advice to patients. Often the circumstances are less than ideal, because patients are anxious, in pain, or feeling unwell. Also, there may be very little time available in which to impart information, as in a busy surgery or outpatient clinic, and therefore all the more reason to present it in the clearest possible way, thereby ensuring the greatest understanding and retention.

All the basic communication skills already discussed in Chapters 9 and 10, and the principles of effective teaching in this chapter, are important. In addition, there are some particular strategies which have been found to be helpful in patient education.[7]

Say Important Things First

Patients are more likely to remember what was said at the beginning of a session, so give the important advice and instructions first, if possible.

Stress and Repeat the Key Points

Patients are more likely to remember what they consider to be important so make sure they realize what the really important points are. For example, say:

"The *most important* thing for you to remember today is . . ."
"The one thing it's *essential* to do is . . ."

Repetition of key points also helps people to remember them.

Give Specific, Precise Advice

Sometimes it is appropriate to give general guidance, but specific, precise advice is more likely to be remembered than vague guidance. For example, say: "I advise you to lose five pounds in the next month" rather than "I advise you to lose weight"; say "Try to take an hour's rest with your feet up every afternoon" rather than "Get more rest".

Other key points which have already been discussed are:
—structure information into categories
—avoid jargon and long words and sentences
—use visual aids, leaflets, handouts and written instructions
—avoid saying too much at once
—ensure that advice is relevant and realistic in the patient's circumstances
—get feedback from the patient to ensure that he understands.

The following exercise is designed to facilitate practice in the skills of patient education we have discussed here and it incorporates basic communication skills (see Chapters 9 and 10).

Exercise — Skills of patient education

Work in groups of three, taking each role in turn.

The *first person* takes the role of the health professional. She selects the topic to be taught, drawing on her own experience, and tells the "patient" his medical history before role-play starts.

The *second person* plays the patient. This patient has one of the following sets of characteristics:
— intelligent, but with very limited understanding of spoken English, no ability to read or write English, and no-one available to translate;
— extremely worried, tense and anxious about his medical condition and prognosis;
— low level of intelligence, barely literate, finds great difficulty in understanding and remembering instructions although he tries hard to be co-operative.

The *third person* takes the role of the observer, using the observer's checklist below.

Role-play the scene in which the health educator is teaching the patient for ten minutes. The observer keeps time. Then give constructive feedback as follows:
— firstly, the "health professional" assesses herself, saying what she felt she did well, and identifying points she feels the need to work on in the future.
— secondly, the "patient" describes how it felt to be the patient, identifying what the health professional did or said which made him feel at ease/put down/anxious/reassured/more confused, and so on.
— finally, the observer gives feedback using the checklist as a guide.

Communication checklist
1. Non-verbal aspects of communication
    eg. tone of voice, posture, gestures, facial expression, use of touch
2. Sequence and structure of key points
    eg. important things first, logical sequence, information in categories
3. Choice of language
    eg. appropriately simple and short, use of jargon/idioms, medical terms
4. Two-way communication
    eg. encourage patient to talk and express feelings, get feedback about how much is understood, open/closed/biassed/multiple questions
5. Amount of information
    eg. too much or too little
6. Clarity of objective(s)
7. Use of repetition
8. Use of emphasis to stress important points

continued on next page

continued

> 9. Any assumptions made but not checked
>   eg. about previous knowledge, facilities for carrying out instructions,
>   willingness to comply
> 10. Anything else?

Another useful way of learning to improve communication skills is to videotape and analyse an interview with a patient.[8]

Teaching Practical Skills

Health professionals are often called upon to teach practical skills, such as relaxation or keep-fit exercises, how to bath a baby or change a nappy, and how to give an injection or to test urine.

All the communication skills we have discussed are relevant, but a few additional points are useful. Teaching a skill is not just about achieving "knowing" and "doing" objectives; that is, it is not *solely* concerned with giving the client information and teaching him new practical skills. It is also necessary to pay attention to what clients *feel*. If people are afraid to do something because they are worried about looking foolish or doing it incorrectly, they are unlikely to succeed: encouragement and step-by-step progress is needed. Confidence-building is as important a part of the health educator's role as developing practical skills.

In order to develop clients' ability to perform a skilled task, a three-stage approach is most effective, namely:
—demonstrate
—rehearse
—practise

Clients will be watching and listening in stage 1, but they become actively involved in *doing* in stages 2 and 3.

It may be useful to begin by using a dummy, for example, when teaching safe lifting techniques, or to use an orange instead of a person when teaching injection techniques. As skills develop, the techniques can be tried in real life situations (lifting people, for example) and perhaps under more difficult circumstances.

Each individual learner needs to progress at his own pace and build up confidence at each stage. For this reason teaching practical skills needs time and patience, but it is worth the investment to get the right skills programme from the beginning. People who have lost confidence in their ability to do something are even more difficult to help than a new learner.

Notes, References and Further Reading

1 For further reading on teaching and learning, see:
   Hills P (1979) *Teaching and Learning as a Communication Process.* London:

Croom Helm. (Includes clear, brief accounts of communication theory and psychology of learning.)

Brown G (1975) *Micro-teaching.* London: Methuen. (Includes exercises on giving information.)

Brown G (1979) *Lecturing and Explaining.* London: Methuen

2 One study found that the use of this technique improved patients' recall by 17%:

Ley P, Bradshaw P W, Eaves D & Walker C M (1973) A method for increasing patients' recall of information presented by doctors. *Psychol Med*, **3**, 217–220

3 For further reading on giving talks (not in a health context, but still useful) see:

Stanton N (1982) *The Business of Communicating.* London: Pan Books, Chs 7 & 8

Jay A (1970) *Effective Presentation.* Management Publications Ltd, for the British Institute of Management

Hasling J (1976) *The Audience, The Message, The Speaker.* New York: McGraw Hill

4 For some evidence about how much patients forget, or do not understand, what they are told, see:

Ley P (1977) Psychological studies of doctor-patient communication. In Rachman S (ed) *Contributions to Medical Psychology.* Oxford: Pergamon Press

Ley P *et al* (1976) Improving doctor-patient communications in general practice. *J Roy Coll Gen Practit*, **26**, 720–724

5 Ley P (1979) The psychology of compliance. In Oborne D, Gruneberg M M & Eiser J R (eds) *Research in Psychology and Medicine.* London: Academic Press

6 Sackett D & Snow J (1979) The magnitude of compliance and non-compliance. In Haynes R B, Taylor D W & Sackett D L (eds) *Compliance in Health Care.* Baltimore: Johns Hopkins University Press

7 This section is based on material in:

Ewles L & Shipster P (1981) *One-to-One Health Education.* East Sussex Area Health Authority.
(Now available from the South East Thames Regional Health Authority, Press and Public Relations Office, Thrift House, Collington Avenue, Bexhill-on-Sea, East Sussex TN39 3NQ.)

8 For information about tape-recording and analysing an interview with a patient, see:

Perkins E R & Anderson D C (1981) *Self-assessment in the National Health Service.* Nafferton Books

Anderson D (1979) Talking with patients about their diet. In Anderson D (ed) *Health Education in Practice.* London: Croom Helm

Chapter 14
Working
Collectively

Summary

This chapter begins with the identification of what working collectively means
in practice, and defining terms. Four ways of working collectively are
discussed, with illustrative examples: campaign work, work with voluntary
organisations, work initiated within statutory agencies, and work with self-help
groups. This is followed by a suggested framework for planning and taking
part in collective action, and a planning exercise.

So far, the PRACTICE part of this book has been concerned with the skills and
methods a health educator uses when working with individual clients or with groups
of clients. A factor common to these approaches is that the health professional, not
the consumer, identifies the people requiring health education and largely takes the
initiative and organisational responsibility.

In contrast, we focus here on ways of working in which the consumers themselves
have more control, through programmes involving whole communities and through
partnerships between health professionals and consumers. We also describe examples
of successful activities which were initiated and directed by consumers themselves
and which gained the support of some health professionals. We have called this
involvement or partnership between consumers and professionals "working
collectively". We discuss ways of working collectively through campaigns, voluntary
organisations, statutory agencies and self-help groups, and explore the opportunities
that exist for collective work between health professionals and consumers.[1]

What Does Working Collectively Mean?

Underlying Beliefs

If working collectively is to be effective it is important to understand what the method
implies. It is based on underlying beliefs about the appropriate response to inequalities
in health.[2] If health professionals become involved, there is no denying that the work
is political, because it means working towards greater equality and social justice. It
means working with people who experience powerlessness and inequality as part

of their everyday lives, and working towards a redistribution of resources and power.

Collective action means working for change, but change determined by consumers, rather than solely by professionals. There are degrees of possible involvement of the consumers. It may be considered as a continuum with power completely in the hands of the professionals at one end, and power completely in the hands of the consumer at the other:

Professional power ————————————————➤ **Consumer power**

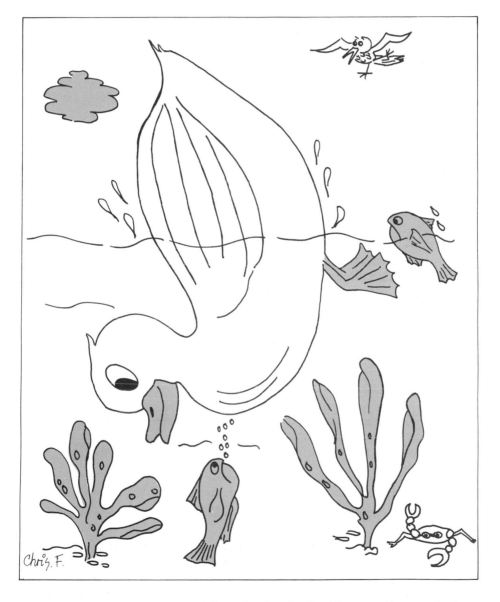

Projects which are consumer-led may be thought of as "bottom-up" approaches!

Different projects work at different points along this continuum. In general, more active participation by consumers means more consumer power. "Top-down" approaches, which are initiated and sustained by professionals are near the left-hand end of this continuum. Projects which are consumer initiated and led are near the right-hand end, and may be thought of as "bottom-up" approaches.

Any form of collective action requires energy, professional humility, patience and time. It challenges the view that only health professionals have the answers to health problems and issues. This is clearly not true, and working alongside consumers gives them a legitimate say in the work, and requires the health professionals to listen.

This may seem a daunting task, but the pay-off may be that:

—clients gain in confidence and experience because they have achieved something for themselves. This encourages self-empowerment and self-esteem. ("I'm OK" in the terms used in the section *Understanding yourself and your clients* in Chapter 9. See also the section *Exploring relationships with clients* in Chapter 8);

—health professionals will have more accurate information about what people want and how people can achieve change;

—health professionals become more accessible to local people, so that the skills and knowledge of both can be more readily available to the other.

Terms Used

Working collectively involves working with communities, but many different terms are used to describe the kinds of activity involved. These terms include "community development", one that has recently come into frequent use in health education,[3] community work and community action. However, there is a problem in that these terms mean different things to different people, so some working definitions may be helpful.

Community A community may be thought of as a network of people. The link between them may be where they live (the X area community), the work they do (the mining community), their ethnic background (the Asian community) or other factors which people have in common. The networks may be formal or informal, but the important point to note in the context of working collectively is that communities have *a capacity to respond* to health issues.

Community work This term is used to describe the work done by a paid worker (a community worker), as distinct from the voluntary activities of the public. It involves working with community groups and organisations to overcome the community's problems and improve their conditions of life. Community work aims to enhance the sense of solidarity and competence in the community.

Community development This term is often used to mean community work, as we have defined it above. However, it includes activities which are not problem-focused, and aims to develop the potential of a community rather than expose its weaknesses. It is often used to describe the planning and political aspects of community work.

Community action This is action which takes place in a locality, initiated by local people in response to a local issue. It often takes place without the involvement of a paid worker.

We now turn to ways of working collectively with communities, which may involve doing community work, or community development work, and may involve community action. The following examples suggest ways by which health professionals and consumers can work together to promote health. Work is mainly focused around a particular issue or within a particular locality. The overriding factor which determines the commitment of participants is the *relevance* of the health issue; it must affect them in some way. Ideology alone is unlikely to motivate.

Campaign Work

Campaigns focus on particular issues, and may be a response to an expressed need or the means of raising awareness of a health issue. Sometimes campaigns are localized and small-scale, but there are many examples of large-scale national health education campaigns, professionally-run with large budgets. They may not always embody the spirit of "working collectively". Some are definitely "top-down" and initiated solely by professionals, such as vaccination campaigns, although some members of the public may feel strongly about the issue and lend the campaign their support.

Health professionals have also been successfully involved with groups of people who campaign for social and political change. One example is their involvement in promoting non-smoking policies for health authorities through the voluntary organisation *Action on Smoking and Health* (ASH), a national body which aims to promote non-smoking.[4] The active support of medical practitioners and health service administrators for this aspect of ASH's work is, no doubt, partly responsible for the increased interest of health authorities in the development of health promotion policies. This is an example of promoting social and political change at *local* level through the development of local policies.

At national level, the newly-formed campaigning body *Triple A* (Action on Alcohol Abuse) is promoting social and political change by, for example, directly lobbying Members of Parliament. Areas in which Triple A will press for action include implementation of a health-based taxation policy, more rigorous enforcement of the law against drinking and driving, and substantially increased funding for health education on the dangers of alcohol. Triple A is backed by the King's Fund and has the support of the Royal Medical Colleges.[5]

Three more examples illustrate what can be achieved in campaign work, and what part the health educator can play.

Group Against Smoking in Public (GASP) is a campaigning group of lay and professional people based in Bristol, whose activities have led to an increase in the provision of no-smoking areas in local restaurants and to the curtailment of tobacco sponsorship of sports and cultural events.[6] In this case, the health professionals involved supplied detailed knowledge of the effect of smoking on the health of smokers and non-smokers and worked with lay people to obtain publicity and policy changes. The recent abolition of smoking on all Underground trains in London illustrates the impact of this kind of campaign and the way in which politicians have also taken it up.

The Campaign for Lead-free Air (CLEAR) seeks to raise public awareness and exert pressure on the government about the need for lead-free air, and was one influence which led to the introduction of new legislation to control the level of lead in petrol.[7] CLEAR has made extensive use of the media for putting across its message. Health professionals can become involved by bringing this publicity to the attention of the widest possible audience, and encouraging a debate to take place.

The Tyne Tees Alcohol Education Campaign started in the north-east of England (the Tyne Tees television area) in 1974, and still exists in 1984. Funded by the Health Education Council, it is run by a regional committee of District Medical Officers, Health Education Officers and representatives of the North East Council on Alcoholism, the Regional Treatment Unit and the Health Education Council. Its aims are to help people to recognize their drinking problems and seek help, and to promote sensible drinking. The campaign strategy includes education and training for field workers, and education for the general public through radio, television, press, exhibitions, talks and workshops.[8] Unlike many other campaigns, it has been carefully and extensively evaluated, and the report makes recommendations on the conditions necessary for conducting successful health education campaigns with large populations.[9] These highlight:

—the need for extensive and intensive systematic research in the community before a campaign is designed. This ensures that the campaign is relevant to the health needs of the population, and takes account of their beliefs, values, attitudes and way of life. For example, it is critical to establish what the usual drinking patterns are: alcohol education geared to drinking spirits is irrelevant in a predominantly beer-drinking population.
—the need to establish support services before the campaign starts. Alcohol advisory centres, for example, should be adequately staffed with trained workers and volunteers before media advertising leads to a flood of enquiries.
—the need to incorporate procedures for monitoring and evaluation at the planning stage; they should not be left to the end when base-line data is no longer available for comparison.
—the need for training front-line workers as health educators. For example, health visitors and social workers are likely to be key educators with the public, but may need training in alcohol education. A training manual was produced, and key tutors were trained.[10] These key tutors, who were health education officers, other professionals and specialist alcohol workers, then trained others to work as alcohol educators and develop local alcohol education programmes. The aim was both to educate the community about alcohol and to turn as many members of the community as possible into active alcohol educators. The training involved participation by group members in order to break down the expert-student relationship and develop confidence in the skills of alcohol education.
—the need for effective communication links between all those involved and for a campaign co-ordinator to play a key role in establishing and maintaining these links.

—the need for clarity and precision in the definitions of the roles and functions of all the organisations involved.

These recommendations are useful principles on which to base campaign work of this type, and they show how health professionals can be involved.

Work with Voluntary Organisations

Voluntary organisations are a response to live issues and problems, such as poverty or loneliness. In the past they often complemented statutory services, but the balance of resources between statutory and voluntary services changes with the political and economic climate. For example, in 1984 in Bristol, a large number of preventive services for children and families are being developed by voluntary organisations such as *Barnardo's* and the *National Children's Home*, at the request and with the financial backing of the local authority.

At national and local levels there are co-ordinating bodies for voluntary organisations. In each area there is a local Council for Voluntary Service or a Council for Community Service, which provides information about local voluntary organisations. They may help volunteers who wish to formalize their activities by creating an organisation and perhaps to attract funds. Nationally, the *National Council for Voluntary Organisations* acts as a co-ordinating body[11] and has produced a handbook for voluntary groups who want to play an active part in promoting health, and a directory of community health initiatives.[12]

An important aspect of health education is providing information about the range of health services available, and helping people to exercise their choice. A number of Community Health Councils and voluntary organisations have undertaken local surveys of health services which not only provide information which is unavailable elsewhere, but may also act as catalysts to bring about improvements in health services.[13] Two examples will illustrate the impact that voluntary organisations can have, and how health professionals can work alongside them.[14]

The National Childbirth Trust (NCT) has been teaching pregnant women for over a quarter of a century, and now has some 250 branches in the country offering antenatal classes.[15] The teachers are nearly always mothers who have been through the pleasures and problems of parenthood themselves. The approach to teaching is thus much closer to mutual aid than the expert-patient relationship which may prevail in NHS antenatal classes. According to a recent survey, nearly every woman who had joined an NCT class found it very helpful in contrast to only about half among those who had been to NHS classes.[16]

The NCT approach seems to be having an impact on NHS provision, with prospective parents being encouraged to make legitimate demands about the birth of their child. Health professionals in the NHS have begun to redefine their ideas about education for childbirth and parenthood, and in some places the NCT provides classes for prospective parents in collaboration with health professionals on health service premises.

Patient participation groups involve lay volunteers working with health professionals in the primary health care team. There are now about 55 patient participation groups and the National Association for Patient Participation in General Practice acts as a co-ordinating body.[17] These groups, mainly based at health centres and group practices, are composed of patients, doctors and other medical staff who come together to discuss their services and how they can be most sensitive to people's needs. They usually put great emphasis on health education to improve patients' own self-care. The Royal College of General Practitioners encourages the patient participation movement, and the initiative to develop a group usually comes from GPs.

These groups show how health professionals and consumers can work in partnership, with patients having a real part to play in the policy and planning of their health services. Supporting such ventures is clearly a vital role for health professionals.

Work Initiated within Statutory Agencies

As we have discussed, one of the principles of "working collectively" is the encouragement of lay people to have more say in the response to health issues. Taken to its logical conclusion, this means that professional health educators should work towards making themselves redundant! However, there are many initiatives which both start and remain within statutory services, and we will discuss these now.

There are contradictions in this approach, because control is retained in the hands of professionals. Transferring power into the hands of consumers causes tension for the health professional which may include having to address the following questions:

— does identifying with local people mean taking a stand against colleagues and their practice? (For example, local people may complain about the services at their health clinic, and wish to initiate changes.)
— does a lay interpretation of health issues demean a professional view? (For example, lay people may campaign for more high-technology medical facilities, whereas the professional, with a greater knowledge of the potential for prevention, may believe that resources should be allocated to preventive work.)
— will the health professional's manager be happy that she should devote time to activities that could lead to criticism of health services? (For example, working with ethnic minorities may reveal racist attitudes in health service staff.)

These are not new tensions, but working collectively within the health services brings them into sharper focus (see also Chapter 4 *Ethical Aspects of Health Education*).

An example of a project initiated by professionals is the *Riverside Child Health Project* on Tyneside.[18] Two community workers work alongside a health visitor and local GPs. The medical staff encouraged the involvement of lay people in running the project, and recognizing the key role played by the community workers who could communicate well with members of the local community and bridge the gap between health professionals and lay people.

A health project in Peckham focused on making health information available to local people and increasing their confidence in managing their own health. An account of this project shows that it declined when the community worker left.[19] The project could be seen as a failure in that it was obviously dependent on the community worker and on outside sources of funding. The community failed to develop lay leadership to carry on in the absence of a professional helper, illustrating the difficulties of transferring control. However, if the project is seen as a time-limited educational exercise to enable members to take increased responsibilities for their health and to use health services more effectively then it was a success.

Work with Self-help Groups

Self-help groups can be defined as groups of people who feel that they have a common problem and have joined together to do something about it.[20] Within this broad definition self-help groups cover a very wide range of problems and activities: they may focus on medical, behavioural or social problems, and there appears to be no such thing as a typical self-help group.[21] In general, most people who have joined a self-help group feel that their involvement has been of benefit to them, and some feel that they have benefited from the opportunity to help others.

Perhaps the most well-known self-help group is *Alcoholics Anonymous*,[22] which operates throughout much of the world. Small, local self-help groups may also flourish. For example, the advantages of mutual aid have been used by a Harlow health visitor to initiate a network of post-natal support groups called CHAT (*Contact, Health and Teaching*). Local mothers act as group leaders and draw on the help of others in the network in undertaking health education.[23]

In general, self-help groups aim to provide one or more of the following:

1 information and advice;
2 mutual emotional support for people "in the same boat";
3 direct services to help members to cope with their problems;
4 a range of social activities;
5 pressure-group activities to increase public awareness of their problems, lobby for improved services where appropriate, and change attitudes towards people with problems.

Self-help mushroomed in the UK in the 70s and many writers show a tendency to view it as a panacea for all ills.[24] But in reality, a viable self-help group is not easy to establish and run. A survey of local self-help groups undertaken by Merton, Sutton and Wandsworth Health Education Unit showed that many groups had very limited opening times, some groups were doing little more than handing out literature and many groups were short-lived and left no forwarding address.[25]

A report of the *Mind Yourself* project, which aimed to stimulate the development of self-help for mental health, is illuminating. The project worker writes: "During the first year of the project's existence I quickly learned the hard way that there was more to setting up a self-help group than getting like-minded people together in a cosy room with a kettle and a packet of tea bags".[26]

She identifies the difficulties experienced by members in being able to function as a self-help group as the same difficulties that brought people into the group in the first place, namely:
—low self-esteem;
—lack of assertiveness;
—inability to feel deeply;

—inability to trust anyone;
—difficulty in making close relationships.

These difficulties were overcome by using a variety of exercises, and the following factors seemed to be critical:
—*structure:* groups are more successful if helpers take an active role in structuring them;
—*support:* groups need long-term support, perhaps indefinitely;
—*self-help therapy:* groups need to be taught self-help exercises and techniques;
—*a course for leaders,* Skills of Self-help, was devised.

   Self-help, as applied in this successful project, is a far cry from simple mutual aid, and seems to have more in common with social skills training.
   The involvement of a health professional with a self-help group requires that she should understand what it has taken for these people to come together. A tremendous amount of encouragement may be required to prevent a group from folding up, particularly in the early stages. People may have very little confidence in their own abilities to take action, to offer support, to write letters or to begin a discussion, for example, and they may easily give up because of the daunting nature of the task. Professionals may be able to function well in these kinds of activities, and it is all too easy to take over or subtly denigrate the efforts of individuals or groups.
   The ways by which health professionals can work with self-help groups may be summarized as:
—initiating and stimulating the development of new groups;
—helping a group to set out achievable early targets, so that they are quickly operating from a position of success;
—giving continuous encouragement without taking over;
—providing professional help on request, such as advice to individuals or talks to groups;
—providing financial support;
—providing other resources such as rooms, leaflets or copying facilities;
—publicising groups and referring new members to them.

Working Collectively—Which Approach

Some of the examples we have discussed are client-directed, and some are professionally-led. Some focus on the need for particular members of the community to help themselves, whereas others focus on the need for social and political change on a particular issue. Many contain elements related to all these dimensions.
   In terms of the health education approaches discussed in Chapter 3, activities which focus on helping and educating individuals reflect medical, behaviour change or educational approaches. Activities which focus on social or political change reflect the social change approach. In both cases, activities may be client-directed or professionally-led.

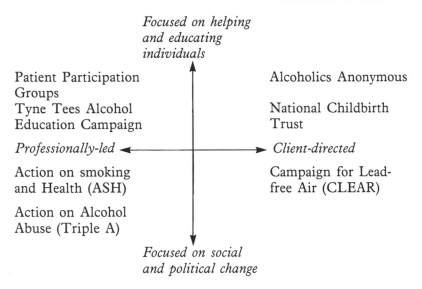

*Focused on helping
and educating
individuals*

Patient Participation
Groups
Tyne Tees Alcohol
Education Campaign

Alcoholics Anonymous

National Childbirth
Trust

Professionally-led ◄──────────► *Client-directed*

Action on smoking
and Health (ASH)

Campaign for Lead-
free Air (CLEAR)

Action on Alcohol
Abuse (Triple A)

*Focused on social
and political change*

A Framework for Collective Action

A framework for planning and taking part in collective action has been developed
for and by community workers. It can also be helpful to health professionals who
wish to become more involved in community-based health education, working with
lay people in the ways we have already discussed. The framework identifies nine
major tasks, and we have interpreted each task in a health education context.[27]

1 Planning and Consulting

You might be the first person to have thought about an issue, but this is most unlikely;
therefore, planning should involve deciding who to consult and conveying as much
information as possible to other interested parties. The example of the Alcohol
Education Campaign discussed previously highlights the need for work to begin *before*
the action starts. For example, if you want to improve the poor access to health services
offered to Asian patients in your locality, the first contact might be with the local
Council for Racial Equality (CRE). This could save much time and difficulty by
obtaining clear information about the current provision of services within that
community from people who are closely involved. The local CRE could also identify
the most appropriate people to speak to in that community.

2 Getting to Know the Community

It is important not to rely solely on professional perceptions, which often stem from
a problem-centred view of a locality; for example, police will talk about crime, social
workers about numbers of children in care. Local newspapers are a useful source
of information about the needs, interests and activities of a locality, and local
newspapers may have a library service which will select material on a particular issue
over the previous five years. Another approach is to *walk* — not drive — around the

neighbourhood. Groups of young people on street corners, smells from fast-food shops, and the range and price of goods in shop windows can reveal a lot about local life-style and socio-economic status (see also the section *Identifying health education needs* in Chapter 6).

3 Working Out What to do Next

The information you acquire will enable you to decide whether or not your original concern is justified, how to use the information and what to do next. For example, are you going to respond to the issue by involving consumers from the start? Are you going to involve colleagues, and what support can you expect? It might be useful to write down what you have done so far and seek the impartial views of someone who has not been involved.

4 Making Contacts and Bringing People Together

Many contacts may already have been made, and people who have a common interest or experience may have been identified. For example, you might have come across many people who have said that they would like to help others to avoid their bad experience following a bereavement, the birth of a handicapped child or a hysterectomy. By bringing them together, you may find that the collective energy of a group generates ideas for future action and you can begin to share the work. This means that your role may also begin to change, from being an initiator to being a supporter.

5 Forming and Building Organisations

The group of people you have brought together may be hesitant about taking action and encouraging others to join. The necessary administrative work may put them off, so you may have to help them to understand the costs and benefits of formalizing the group. The advantages of having a formal organisation are that it can apply for financial help and for recognitition as a legitimate body; the disadvantages might be that control could be exercised from outside, or that members are attracted who turn out to be more of a hindrance than a help. The local Council for Voluntary Service can be an extremely useful contact since it provides a helpful service for newly-formed groups, and affiliation to the Council brings credibility in itself.

6 Helping to Clarify Goals and Priorities

It is frequently difficult to decide whether the goals and priorities of the group are those of the people you are working with, or your own. For example, a group of women who have had a hysterectomy and are concerned at the lack of information and help they were given may wish to campaign for better support from their own doctor. But *you* may wish instead to raise the issue with the Community Health Council in order to obtain more broadly based action. Is it your campaign or theirs?

Exercise — Planning and taking part in collective action on a health issue

Complete the following statements as far as you can, as a planning exercise:

The issue is . . .
The people I need to talk to are . . .
The documents I need to read are . . .
I can get to know more about the community by . . .
The information that is likely to be available is . . .
I intend to look for this information by . . .
Work done on this issue elsewhere is . . .
The people who are likely to be supportive are . . .
The people I should avoid offending are . . .
The period of time I can spend on this issue is . . .
The amount of time I can give it during this period is . . .
The person I will talk to in order to work out what to do next is . . .

---

7 Keeping the Organisation Going

With the passage of time, people may lose their enthusiasm. You may be able to provide additional impetus by having the advantage of being involved as part of your paid work. You need to be sensitive to the many ways by which an organisation can lose its way, and you may be able to help, in such circumstances, by:
— discovering what similar activities are taking place elsewhere and circulating details to members of the organisation;
— drawing the issue to the attention of the district health authority, and conveying the response to the group;
— helping the group to produce their own health education materials such as posters, leaflets or even a videotape, and distributing them;
— looking at other health education material on the topic;
— encouraging members of the group to talk about their work to other people, such as groups of interested professionals and students;
— circulating everyone to remind them of meetings;
— providing practical support such as photocopying or typing;
— introducing new members.

8 Dealing with Friends and Enemies

The issue you are concerned with will probably have a local history, and be likely to have both lost and won support in the past. You need to identify other interest groups, and work with the group in deciding how to tackle them. For instance, you need to win friends in the local Licensed Victuallers Association before you run an alcohol education campaign because lack of their support could mean that you will have to fight a powerful lobby.

Careful preparation, even rehearsal, can help a group to avoid being unevenly matched in a dialogue with people who are used to confronting others and to negotiating at meetings.[28]

9 Leavings and Endings

There comes a point when your involvement has to stop, maybe because you change your job or the priorities of your work, or because the group is now self-sufficient. Occasionally, you and the group may need to recognize that you have done all that you can do, and that doing any more would be flogging a dead horse.

Ending your involvement provides the opportunity for a final evaluation of what has been achieved for the consumer, what your own contribution has been, where the issues can be taken in the future and who might be involved.

Notes, References and Further Reading

1   For further reading on lay participation in health promotion and health care, see:

McEwen J, Martini C J M & Wilkins N (1983) *Participation in Health*. London: Croom Helm

2   For further reading on inequalities in health, and the implications for action, see:

Townsend P & Davidson N (1982) *Inequalities in Health*. Harmondsworth: Penguin Books

Doyal L & Pennell I (1979) *The Political Economy of Health*. London: Pluto Press

Mitchell J (1984) *What is to be done about Illness and Health?* Harmondsworth: Penguin Books

3   See, for example:

Hubley J (1980) Community development and health education. *J Inst Hlth Educ*, 18, 113–120

4   See: Olsen N D L, Roberts J & Castle P (1981) *Smoking Prevention: a Health Promotion Guide for the NHS*. An ASH handbook, published by, and available from, ASH, 5 Mortimer Street, London W1

5   Action on Alcohol Abuse, 26 Craven Street, London WC2. Triple A has representatives from the Royal Colleges of General Practitioners, Physicians and Psychiatrists, all the other Medical Royal Colleges, and Faculty of Community Medicine and the Health Education Council.

6   Naidoo J (1983) GASP—a new anti-smoking initiative. *J Inst Hlth Educ*, 21, (1)

Report (1984) AGHAST, GASP and the right ANSR. In "Notes and News", *Lancet*, 30 July

7   For further reading about campaigning, written by the director of CLEAR see:

Wilson D (1984) *Pressure: the A-Z of Campaigning in Britain*. London: Heinemann

8 For further discussion of this campaign, see:

Simnett I (1983) A personal perspective on the Tyne Tees Alcohol Education Campaign. *J Inst Hlth Educ*, 21 (2)

9 The evaluation report, available from the Health Education Council, is:

Budd J, Gray P & McCron R (1982) *The Tyne Tees Alcohol Education Campaign— an Evaluation.* Centre for Mass Communication Research, Leicester University

10 Simnett K I, Wright L & Evans M (1983) *Drinking Choices—a Training Manual for Alcohol Educators.* London: Health Education Council/TACADE

11 National Council for Voluntary Organisations, 26 Bedford Square, London WC1B 3HU

12 Smith C (1982) *Community-based Health Initiatives—a Handbook for Voluntary Groups.* National Council for Voluntary Organisations

Smith C & Lacey M (1982) *Directory of Community Health Initiatives.* National Council for Voluntary Organisations

Allen R & Purkis A (1983) *Health in the Round: Voluntary Action and Ante-natal Services.* National Council for Voluntary Organisations

13 See, for example:

Waltham Forest District Community Health Council (1981) *Having a Baby Second Time Round.* Waltham Forest CHC

14 For more examples in the field of preventive health care in pregnancy and early childhood see:

Dowling S (1983) *Health for a Change.* Child Poverty Action Group, in Association with the National Extension College, Chapter 8.
(This book is a comprehensive review of new developments in the way preventive health care in pregnancy and early childhood is provided, and discusses over 60 schemes in England and Wales.)

15 National Childbirth Trust, 9 Queensborough Terrace, London W2 3TB

16 Boyd C & Sellers L (1982) *The British Way of Birth.* London: Pan Books

17 National Association for Patient Participation in General Practice, c/o Whiteladies Health Centre, Whatley Road, Bristol BS8 2PN
Further reading on patient participation:

Klein R (1984) Patient participation—much like an elastic stocking. *Health Soc Serv J*, 5 January, 20

Shearer A (1983) The patient revolution in Kentish Town, *Self Health*, (1) November

18 The Riverside project is described in:

Smith C (1982) *Community Based Health Initiatives—a Handbook for Voluntary Groups.* National Council for Voluntary Organisations

19 Fisher B H & Cochrane M (1982) Peckham Health Project—raising health consciousness. *Br Med J*, **1**, 1843–1845

20 This definition is used in:

Richardson A & Goodman M (1983) *Self-help and Social Care—mutual Aid Organisations in Practice.* Policy Studies Institute, London.
(This report includes an extensive discussion of alternative definitions of self-help groups.)

21 For further reading on self-help groups in health, see:

Robinson D & Henry S (1977) *Self-help and Health.* Oxford: Martin Robertson

Robinson D & Robinson Y (1979) *From Self-Help to Health.* London: Concord Books

Hatch S & Kickbusch I (eds) (In press) *Involvement in Health: Self-help and Self-care in Europe.* London: Croom Helm

22 Robinson D (1979) *Talking out of Alcoholism: the Self-help Process of Alcoholics Anonymous.* London: Croom Helm

23 Hiskins G (1981) How mothers help themselves. *Health Visitor*, **53** (3), 108–111

24 Levy I (1982) Mutual support groups in Great Britain: a survey. *Soc Sci Med*, **16**, 1265–1275

25 Webb P (1983) Ready, willing but able? *J Roy Soc Hlth*, **1**, 35–41

26 Hawkins G (1982) Self-help in Leeds. In *Working Together? Voluntary and Statutory Mental Health Services.* A report of MIND's 1982 Annual Conference, MIND Publications

27 Material in this section is based on:

Henderson P & Thomas D N (1980) *Skills in Neighbourhood Work.* National Institute of Social Services Library, No. 39. London: George Allen & Unwin
Reproduced by permission of the authors and their publishers

A videotape *Learning more about Community Work* illustrates the nine tasks we discuss. It is available from: National Institute of Social Work, 5 Tavistock Place, London WC1 9SS

For additional further reading, see:

Twelvetrees A (1982) *Community Work.* London: British Association of Social Work/Macmillan

Boot N (1984) *Promoting Health with Community Groups.* Nottingham Practical Papers in Health Education No 10. University of Nottingham Department of Adult Education/Nottinghamshire Health Education Unit. Available from the Health Education Unit, Huntingdon House, Huntingdon Street, Nottingham, NG1 3LZ

28 For useful guidelines on how to negotiate, see:

Brewster C (1984) *Understanding Industrial Relations.* London: Pan Books, Ch 8

Chapter 15
Working
with the
Mass Media

Summary

The chapter starts by identifying the variety of ways in which the mass media are channels of health education, followed by a discussion on what they can be expected to achieve and how they can be used effectively. The chapter then concentrates on giving practical help to health professionals working with television, radio and local press. There are exercises on preparing and presenting material on television and radio, writing a press release and a "letter to the editor".

The mass media are the channels of communication to large numbers of people: television, radio, magazines and newspapers, books, displays and exhibitions.[1]

Health messages are conveyed through the mass media in a number of different ways:
—planned deliberate health promotion, eg. displays and exhibitions on health themes, Health Education Council advertisements on television and in newspapers, Open University community education programmes on health;
—health promotion by advertisers and manufacturers of "healthy" products, eg. advertisements for wholemeal bread or for toothpaste, educational leaflets on "feeding your baby" or "slimming" which also promote relevant products;
—books, documentaries and articles about health issues, eg. television programmes and magazine articles about diet, pollution or fitness;
—discussion of health issues as a by-product of news items or entertainment programmes, notably soap-opera serials where a character has a health problem;
—health (or anti-health) messages conveyed covertly, eg. well-known personalities or fictional characters refusing cigarettes or, conversely, chain-smoking;
—planned promotion of anti-health messages (probably denied or rationalized as not anti-health!), eg. advertisements for sweets and chocolates.

Health professionals are most likely to become involved in working with the mass media when undertaking programmes of planned health promotion, or when health becomes a news item. They may also participate in the production of documentary programmes and articles, particularly for local radio and newspapers.

Using the Mass Media for Health Education

The mass media can reach an enormous number of people, including people to whom the health professional may not have personal access. However, this is no justification for its indiscriminate use, because many research studies have now shown that the direct persuasive power of the mass media is very limited.[2] Expectations that the mass media *alone* will produce dramatic long-term changes in health behaviour are doomed to disappointment.

Some Difficulties

Mass media messages must be very carefully designed so that the right message gets to the target audience in a form appropriate to their needs and lifestyle. Commercial advertising applies in-depth research to the target audience; this has been applied in health education campaigns but it is obviously very costly.[3]

Health education advertising has the additional problem that the audience is often asked to identify with a message that they may find uncomfortable or even threatening (for example, Christmas drinking-and-driving advertisements). The audience will search for ways of rejecting the message, and one inaccurate detail in the portrayal of the lifestyle of the audience could lead to rejection. This means that the images and scenarios require repeated testing on sample potential audiences. To overcome the problem of rejected messages, much current health education advertising takes a positive approach, using emotions and atmosphere to create, for example, a positive image for the non-smoker.

Health education advertising can be an inappropriate response to some problems. The Scottish Health Education Group, for example, in a detailed study of young people's attitudes towards sexual behaviour and contraception, concluded that the main need was for greater communication between young people themselves, and between young people and parents, schools, and society as a whole.[4] Basically, this is an educational problem and the role of the mass media is very limited. The ethical and moral issues involved, and society's changing and conflicting attitudes, cannot be addressed by advertisements. Instead, young people need help in understanding and coping with conflicting pressures.

Another problem in this sensitive area is censorship; an advertisement that might be interpreted as condoning sexual activity in teenagers will almost certainly be censored! Censorship exacerbates what is really a failure of society to permit open, healthy debate on these issues. Radio and television programmes may play a part here, by providing models to show how parents may discuss these issues with their children and through legitimizing sexual behaviour as a topic for discussion.

Achieving Health Education Goals

Properly used, however, the mass media can certainly be a useful channel for health education. The following points summarize what we can reasonably expect to achieve, expressed in terms of the *health education goals* discussed in Chapter 2.

Raising health consciousness The mass media are very useful for drawing the attention of the public to a health issue, which then becomes a matter of public interest and debate. This is sometimes known as "agenda-setting" because it raises the issues which are subsequently discussed, in the same way as a committee meeting agenda identifies the items for the committee's attention. Heart transplants and test-tube babies are examples of health issues which the news media put on the agenda of public debate. These examples also illustrate how the public agenda about health is usually actually about illness and disability, because most reporting of health issues stresses technological expertise and hospital-based curative medicine.[5] Positive health promotion is rarely hot news.

Increasing health knowledge Once a topic is on the public agenda, the mass media can be used to inform the public and stimulate lively debate. Discussion about whooping cough vaccination, fluoridation of water supplies, health service cuts, tobacco sponsorship of sports events and the provision of services for the disabled are examples of areas of informed debate on issues in the public eye in recent years.

Increasing self-awareness and influencing attitude change, decision-making and behaviour change It is not easy to identify the effect of the mass media in these areas, because mass media influences are inextricably bound up with all the other aspects of people's lives which affect their health attitudes and behaviour. However, it is clear that the mass media can be effective in eliciting an *immediate emotional response*, which may lead to an immediate action. An example of this is how people responded to the scare about brain damage caused by whooping cough vaccine by not taking their children to be vaccinated. Another example is the thousands of people who write for leaflets on how to give up smoking after a television programme on the subject. These are *short-term* responses. A permanent change in people's smoking, eating or drinking habits, for example, is unlikely to be achieved as a result of a mass media publicity alone.[6]

As the primary response of people to the mass media is emotional and not rational, it is very important not to raise anxieties irresponsibly. For example, publicity about rubella-damaged babies should always be accompanied by clear, simple and specific advice about the effects of rubella and how these can be avoided.

Deaths blamed on TV

Panorama distorted facts, says expert

By JOHN ILLMAN

BETWEEN 200 and 300 people died prematurely as a result of a TV programme, an eminent medical consultant claimed yesterday.

Dr Christopher Pallis said the BBC's controversial Panorama presentation on brain death in 1980 led to a sharp fall in the number of people prepared to donate their kidneys in the event of sudden death.

He accused the BBC of grossly distorting scientific data in the programme, adding : 'It had a tragic effect on the transplantation programme'

Dr Pallis, consultant neurologist at London's Hammersmith Hospital, was speaking on Medical Disasters in Perspective at the British Association for the Advancement of Science

meeting in Brighton.

Another speaker was Peter Goodchild, the BBC's head of science and features, whose subject was The Whys and Wherefores of The Reporting on So Called Disasters. But after he finished his lecture, Dr Pallis challenged him to explain the BBC's presentation of facts on the screen.

He maintained that matters apparently confirming brain death studies

had been shown between quotation marks -- but in fact the studies had not contained those statements. A BBC executive had said of this practice : 'We often put things in single quotes. That is our summary of what the text means. If it is a genuine quote it goes between double quotation marks.'

Asked if the BBC would continue to 'put things between quotation marks which are not quotes,' Mr Goodchild replied : 'I guess they probably will . . . but when you are quoting, it is normally quite clear, within the context of the programme, that double inverted commas means a quote. The point you are making about the programme is obviously a valid one. It has had a reaction. '

The mass media can be effective in eliciting an immediate emotional response! (Reproduced from the *Daily Mail* of 27 August 1983 by the kind permission of Associated Newspapers Group.)

Effecting social change We have already said that the mass media are effective in raising health consciousness, increasing health knowledge and arousing an immediate emotional response. All these are important for producing a climate of public opinion which will favour social change. An example of a social change was the introduction in 1983 of legislation to enforce the wearing of car seat belts. This legislation was finally enacted after years of "Clunk-click" media advertising and public debate, which *did not* in itself make people wear their seat belts in substantial numbers but helped to produce a climate of public opinion in which legislation was acceptable.[7]

The Mass Media as Part of an Overall Strategy

We have stressed that the mass media *alone* are unlikely to produce dramatic long-term changes in health behaviour; it is essential to realize that the most effective use of the mass media is as part of an overall strategy which includes face-to-face discussion and personal help. For example, mass media publicity about sensible drinking should include information about where to go and who to see if people want help, and, of course, the helping agencies must be fully prepared to give that help.

The following example of a successful American mass media campaign illustrates the effectiveness of the mass media in agenda-setting and informing, and the importance of personal follow-up work by health professionals.

Example — The effective use of the mass media in health education

The Stanford University Heart Disease Prevention Programme[8]

This was an experiment in community behaviour change through education about the risks of cardiovascular disease, which was begun in 1972 in California.

The mass media elements involved exposing the population of the experimental communities to about three hours of television programmes, over fifty television announcements, one hundred radio spot broadcasts, several hours of radio programmes, weekly newspaper columns, newspaper advertisements and stories, posters in buses, stores and worksites, and printed material sent by mail to people's homes.

The research team found that the level of knowledge about risk factors associated with heart disease increased dramatically in the experimental communities and that there were accompanying reductions in saturated fat intake, cigarette smoking, plasma cholesterol levels, systolic blood pressure and the overall probability of contracting heart disease.

When the mass media elements were supplemented by face-to-face instruction not only were the results improved in the short term, but they were maintained over three years.

Creating Opportunities

Health professionals may have misgivings about working with the mass media, particularly with reporters and interviewers in local news media (local newspapers, radio and television). For example, health educators may feel that "They'll misquote me", "I'll dry up if I'm interviewed", "They'll sensationalize the issue" or "I'll get into trouble with my manager".

The basis for these fears is often exaggerated, although there may be a grain of truth in them. The real truth may be that health professionals are scared of the exposure. But journalists in newspapers, radio and television can be very helpful allies, so what can be done to overcome these fears?

A way forward is to establish personal contact with local journalists. Do not wait for them to ring you—you ring them. Establish an informal, personal relationship: get to know how they work and what their special areas of interest are—this will help to develop mutual trust and understanding. You can then approach them if you wish to give exposure to a particular topic, or if you want to discuss how the media are portraying a current issue. The benefits are mutual; journalists will be more likely to approach you to get your help with an item of health news.[9]

The following sections give practical guidelines on working with radio, television and local newspapers. Having this information may also help to overcome fear of working with the news media.

Working with Radio and Television

Using a spot on radio or television effectively requires preparation and skill. The following checklists are prepared for health professionals who find themselves, literally, "on the spot". They cover the three areas where work is needed: finding out about the programme, preparing the message and preparing the presentation.[10]

Finding out about the Programme

—What programme is it? What sort of approach does the programme have? How long is it? When is it to be transmitted? What kind of audience does it have?
—Why is your topic of interest *now:* is there some local or national controversy or news item which sparked off interest? If so, do you know all about it?
—How are you going to be presented: an information spot, an interview or a discussion panel?
  If it is an interview: who will do it? Will it be in the studio, or on location (perhaps in your workplace or outdoors), or "down the line" (where you are in one studio and the interviewer in another)?
  If it is to be a discussion: who else will be taking part?
—Will it be broadcast live or recorded first?
—How much time are you likely to have on the programme?
—When and where is the broadcast or recording to take place?

Preparing the Message

—Do your homework. You may know a lot or a little about the subject, but in either case you need to identify exactly what it is you want to get across, and to have this very clearly in your mind *before* you are "on the air".

—Be positive. Emphasize the good news, *not* a series of don'ts. Tell people what they *can* do and emphasize the benefits.

—You should have two or three key points to put across, and *no more*. You can expand on these and describe them in different ways but do not overload your audience with too much detail or too many points. They will not remember the additional information anyway, and may even forget the key points.

—Use anecdotes and analogies to illustrate what you mean; simple messages do not have to be bald and boring. Tell stories (short ones!) and use real-life experiences. Put complex points over with everyday analogies, eg. "Use too much fertilizer and you'll kill the plants—use the right amount and they'll grow strong and healthy. The same applies to food and people."

—Avoid technical terms (unless these are essential, in which case use them and explain them) and jargon, but do not be patronizing. It helps to pitch the level right if you imagine that you are talking to an intelligent 14-to-15-year-old whom you have never met before.

Presenting Your Message

—Accept that you are nervous and regard it as a good thing because it means that you will be keyed up to do your best. Remember that the interviewer is there to help you tell your story and to put you at ease.

—Perform with more than 100% liveliness and conviction. Be alert and (if you are on television) look alert at all times. Always assume that the camera is on you even when you are not talking. Make sure your eyes look convincing and involved.

—Speak with your normal voice; if you have a regional accent this will make you more interesting to listen to. Speak clearly and distinctly, and (especially on radio) vary the pitch and speed.

—Make sure you say what *you* want to say. You do not have to follow the line of the interviewer's questions if, for good reason, you do not wish to. Provided you stick to the broad framework of agreed subjects, you have every right to steer the interview or discussion in such a way that you get over what you want to say. Regard the questions as springboards from which to make your points. For example, if you do not like a question you can say:

"I can't really answer that question without explaining first that . . ."
"The real problem behind all this is . . ."
"We don't know the answer to that at the moment, but what we do know is . . ."

—When the interview is over, sit still, keep alert and keep quiet until you are *told* it is over.

—On television, wear what makes you feel comfortable and good. Avoid wearing blue or bright red, predominant stripes, small patterns or flashing jewellery. As you will appear as a "talking head" for most of the time, pay special attention to what you wear in the neckline area.

Exercise — Looking good and sounding good on television and radio

1 Prepare your message

Select a health education topic that you are familiar with, eg. slimming, eating health-giving food, sensible drinking, feeding your baby, keeping fit, avoiding home accidents, living with stress.

Identify *three* key points you would want to put across in a five-minute radio or television interview. Be clear in your mind:
— what the three key points are;
— how you will explain them in an interesting way — what illustrations, analogies, or anecdotes you could use;
— how you will develop your points further if you have time.

2 Practise your presentation

Get a partner to act as your interviewer, and record your interview on an audio or a videotape. Ask a third person to be an observer. Play the tape back and assess your performance:
— did you sound/look lively, alert and convincing?
— was your voice clearly understandable? What did it sound like for speed and pitch?
— did you get your key points across? Did you do so in an interesting way?
— were you able to deal with "difficult" questions?

Working with the Local Press

Local newspapers are an excellent medium for health education in the smaller community. Local journalists will be interested in newsworthy health issues and it is worth studying the newspapers to see who writes about health topics; often it is the writers of the Women's Page. When you have something you wish to have published in the paper, get in touch with these particular journalists and try to establish a personal professional relationship.

In addition to giving information personally, it may be helpful to produce a press release, which journalists can then use as the basis for a story in the paper. Obviously it is important that the press release itself is sufficiently interesting to get the attention of a journalist, and taking account of the following points will help.

How to Write a Press Release

1 Put "News Release" or "Press Release" at the top, along with the name of the organisation issuing it and the date.

2 Type it in double spacing, using one side of the paper only, to facilitate any necessary alteration and scissors-and-paste re-makeup by the journalist.
3 Use simple, straightforward, plain English in short sentences (study the sort of language the newspaper usually uses).
4 Give "bullets" of information in short paragraphs.
5 Identify clearly who can be contacted for further information, giving their titles (Dr, Mrs, etc.), first name and surname, and stating who they are, what their address and telephone number is and when they will be available.
6 Include some verbatim quotations (eg. *Mrs Gloria Slim, the District Dietitian, said: "I am delighted at the number of hospitals which now offer patients wholemeal bread on the menu."*).
7 Focus on *people* rather than make generalized statements or quote dry statistics (eg. say: *Last week three Bloggsville children were admitted to the General Hospital after accidentally swallowing weedkiller. This brings to 36 the number who have had treatment this year. Sister Florence Nightingale, in charge of the emergency treatment, said: "It is heartbreaking to see the needless distress this causes . . .".*).
8 Make it *topical*. Refer to recent events, publications, and reports, so that the item is presented as current news and not as a stale repeat of the same old message.
9 Issue your press release so that it arrives at the best time for the paper. For example, Friday or Monday for a weekly paper published on the following Friday is usually best.
10 Give it local relevance. Feature local people and places, not national events.
11 If you run to more than one sheet, always type "More follows" on the bottom of each page. Put "Ends" at the end of the text of the press release.

Example — Press release

BLOGGSHIRE DISTRICT HEALTH AUTHORITY

PRESS RELEASE MAY 30TH 1985

CAMPAIGN TO INCREASE SMEAR TESTS

Bloggsville doctors are worried that so few women are having regular smear tests. They urge that all women over 35 should have a smear test every two years.

Mrs Ethel Bloggs, secretary of Bloggshire Community Health Council, announced today that the Community Health Council is co-operating with doctors, community nurses and health visitors in a campaign to encourage women to have smear tests. The campaign starts today, and will continue throughout June.

continued on next page

continued

Mrs Bloggs said "Smear tests are a quick, painless way of finding out if there are any signs of cancer in the neck of the womb. Finding signs of trouble early means that treatment is easy and effective. Smear tests are available at most health clinics, health centres and doctor's surgeries. We want all women over 35 who haven't had a test in the last two years to have one soon".

Health Visitors will be giving talks about smear tests to over 50 women's clubs in Bloggshire throughout June. There will be special displays and free information leaflets in all clinics, health centres and doctor's surgeries. Mrs Bloggs will join Dr Guy Neegood, the well-known local radio doctor, in his regular "Healthwise" programme on Radio Bloggsville next Thursday, June 5th, at 10.00 am. They will talk about the campaign and explain how women can have the test.

Women are encouraged to phone Bloggsville 123 to make an appointment for a test at their nearest clinic.

—ENDS—

For further information, please contact:

Mrs Ethel Bloggs

Secretary, Bloggshire Community Health Council

Bloggsville General Hospital

Patient's Lane

Bloggsville BV1 2YZ

Telephone: Bloggsville 789

Another way of using the local paper as a medium for health education is by writing letters to the editor. This can keep an issue in the public eye for some time, and provides good opportunities for public debate of controversial issues. Letters to the editor should be short (some newspapers restrict length), to the point and be on one topic only.

Exercise — Writing for the Local Paper

1. Write a press release about a health education issue you are currently concerned about (for example, school meals, uptake of ante-natal classes, glue-sniffing or the local accident black-spot).
2. Write a letter to the editor supporting a current health education campaign, or drawing attention to a specific need for health promotion.

Notes, References and Further Reading

1 For general background reading on the role of the mass media in relation to health and other social issues, see:

Howitt D (1982) *Mass Media and Social Problems.* Oxford: Pergamon Press

2 For discussion of evidence about the effectiveness of mass media in health education, see:

Tones B K (1981) Health education and the misuse of mass media. *J Inst Hlth Educ,* **19** (3)

McCron R & Budd J (1979) Mass communication and health education. In Sutherland I (ed) *Health Education—Perspectives and Choices.* London: George Allen & Unwin, Ch 10

McCron R & Budd J (1981) The role of the mass media in health education: an analysis. In Meyer M (ed) *Health Education by Television and Radio.* Munich: K G Saur Verlag, 118–139

3 Player D A & Leathar D S (1981) Developing socially sensitive advertising. In Leathar D S, Hastings G B & Davies J K (eds) *Health Education and the Media.* Oxford: Pergamon Press, 187–198

4 Bostock Y & Leathar D S (1981) The role of mass media advertising campaigns in influencing attitudes towards contraception among 16–20-year-olds. In Leathar D S, Hastings G B & Davies J K (eds) *Health Education and the Media.* Oxford: Pergamon Press, 45–48

5 Best G, Dennis J & Draper P (1977) *Health, the Mass Media and the National Health Service.* Unit for the Study of Health Policy, Guy's Hospital Medical School, London

6 For example, see:

Raw M & Van de Pligt J (1981) Can television help people stop smoking? In Leathar D S, Hastings G B Davies J K (eds) *Health Education and the Media.* Oxford: Pergamon Press, 387–398

(This is an account of research into the effectiveness of a Granada "Reports Action" programme in 1977. Six hundred thousand people wrote to Granada asking for a free anti-smoking kit. A questionnaire sent to 20,000 of these was

20—EVENING POST, TUESDAY, OCTOBER 26 1982

POSTBAG

Smokers in the firing line for a freedom

THE HEADLINE to S J Whitrow's letter, After Seat Belt Law, Do We Jail The Smokers? (October 19), not only catches our attention but also makes us think.

There is an inescapable logic in the assertion that once you concede that the State has a right to interfere in personal choices to save the individual for his "own good" then there are no constraints on authority from passing restriction of individual behaviour in whatever it deems to be "risky" activities.

Paternalists

Thus having chalked up a victory on compulsory seat belts, the British Medical Association are now pressing harder than ever to bring smoking to an end.

Smokers are in the front of the firing line from these paternalists.

Of course, they are far too subtle to say they seek to ban smoking: they want to restrict personal choice, far more effectively, through the back door — through over-taxation, over-regulation and over-nagging from tax-payer funded health propagandists.

Tide

It is vital to fight for the principle of freedom of choice — to smoke or not — and to arrest the tide of State intervention in this area.

For if the antis win this battle too, they will soon be preparing themselves for the next fight. Like boxing, with the

BMA already showing its hand in campaigning for its prohibition. And like drinking, with former anti-smoking lobbyists now setting up a national body to press for big restrictions on the sale of alcohol.

Even sweets are a target with recent calls for health warnings and no TV adverts before 9 pm!

Rugby

Fatty foods, butter, rugby, motor-cycle scrambling, rock climbing — the list of risky activities which are under threat goes on.

If we value our freedom we must work to defend and extend our personal choice and tell the busybodies, however well intentioned, to mind their own business.

Stephen Eyres
Director
FOREST (Freedom Organisation For The Right To Enjoy Smoking Tobacco), Bondway House, 3-9, Bondway, London SW8 1SJ.

A letter to the editor! (Reproduced by kind permission of the editor, *Bristol Evening Post*)

returned by 12%. This 12% was followed up one year later and of 1,842 people (82%) who replied, 1,809 provided adequate data. Of these, *only 18* people had stopped smoking for at least a year.)

Also see:

O'Byrne D J & Crawley H D (1981) Conquest smoking cessation campaign 1980—an evaluation. In Leathar D S, Hastings G B & Davies J K (eds) *Health Education and the Media*. Oxford: Pergamon Press, 441–453

(A campaign in the Republic of Ireland using press, radio, TV and outdoor posters offered a stop-smoking kit. Follow-up research indicated that 5% of kit recipients had stopped smoking completely three months after the commencement of the campaign. The researchers conclude that the campaign helped in swinging public opinion against smoking, but that it made only a limited contribution as an aid to the would-be non-smoker.)

7   Dillow I, Swann C & Cliff K S (1981) A study of the effect of a health education programme in promoting seat-belt wearing. *Hlth Educ J*, **40** (1)

In 1981, Parliament agreed in principle to the compulsory wearing of seat belts. In 1983, regulations came into force. (Motor Vehicles (Wearing of Seat Belts) Regulations 1982, S.I. 1982, no. 1203.)

8   Maccoby N & Solomon D (1981) Experiments in risk reduction through community health education. In Meyer M (ed) *Health Education by Television and Radio*. Munich: K G Saur Verlag, 140–166

9   For further reading on journalism and working with the media, see:

MacShane D (1979) *Using the Media—How to Deal with the Press, Television and Radio*. London: Pluto Press

Hodgson F W (1984) *Modern Newspaper Practice*. London: Heinemann

10   Further reading on how to survive on television and radio:

Bland M (1979) *You're On Next!* London: Kogan Page

Chapter 16
Using and Producing
Health Education
Materials

Summary

The first part of the chapter suggests some general principles governing the choice of health education materials. This is followed by a summary of the uses, advantages and limitations of the main types of teaching materials and audio-visual aids. The last section in the chapter outlines points for making the most of display materials, for producing written materials and for presenting statistical information. The chapter includes exercises on the "Gobbledygook Test", writing plain English and presenting statistics in visual ways.

Teaching materials and audiovisual aids such as leaflets, posters and films, are used extensively in the practice of health education.[1] But are they always used *effectively?* In this chapter we aim to give the health professional information and guidelines to help her to choose, produce and use materials with maximum effectiveness. We begin with some general principles on the choice of teaching materials and audiovisual aids.

Health Education Materials — Criteria for Choice

The following list of questions is designed to help the health professional to make and select the most appropriate and useful materials for displays, group teaching or use with individual clients.

Are the Materials Ethically Acceptable?

Material that, for example, is scaremongering, over-authoritarian, victim-blaming, sexist or racist, ignores the values and culture of the consumers, raises expectations of health services which cannot be met, or includes advertising of potentially health-demoting products such as confectionery, is ethically unacceptable.

Is the Information Sound?

Is the information in the materials accurate, up-to-date, unbiassed and complete? Or does it contain half-truths, one-sided information on controversial issues, and out-of-date or incomplete messages?

Is it Relevant for the Consumers?

Does it reflect the values and culture of the consumers? Does it reflect their concerns? Does it take into account the age, ethnic group, sex and socio-economic status of the consumers? Does it reflect local practice and conditions and health services available? Obvious examples of irrelevance are films portraying American lifestyles, or homes of relatively affluent families—both irrelevant to working class British consumers.

Will the Consumers Understand it?

Is the information written in plain English which consumers will readily understand? (There is more about writing plain English and assessing readability later in this chapter.) Are there any incorrect assumptions about the level of existing knowledge?

Does it Meet the Specific Aims of Your Health Education?

Are the materials tailored to the particular aims of your teaching? Do they contain the information you want to convey? Is there too much or too little?

Is this the most Appropriate Kind of Material?

Will another kind of teaching aid be better because it is more flexible (eg. will slides be better than a film because they can be edited)? Will something else be cheaper and just as effective (eg. a videotape instead of a film)? Could the real thing be substituted more effectively for a celluloid or artificial version (eg. parents in person talking about their experience of a new baby instead of appearing on film, babies instead of dolls, actual foods instead of pictures or models)?

The Range of Materials—Uses, Advantages and Limitations

There is a wide range of aids available to the health educator, some of which may be more familiar than others. We would like to emphasize two points by way of introduction; the first is that teaching aids are *aids* and not substitutes for the teacher. Films, for example, are easily misused by being presented without an introduction or with no follow-up discussion and shown just because "it is a good film". Secondly, it takes time and practice to become familiar and comfortable with all the aids available, and it takes courage to try out new things—but it is worth it.

The following summary briefly outlines the uses, advantages and limitations of the main types of aid. Further reading for more detailed information is given at the end of this chapter, but reading is no substitute for practice and experiment.[2]

Leaflets, Handouts and Other Written Materials

Uses and Advantages

1 Allows client self-pacing and self-teaching.
2 Consumers can "revise" the content of health teaching at their leisure.
3 Information can be shared with relatives and friends.
4 Can give further details (eg. statistics) which would clutter up a talk.
5 Handouts are easily produced, duplicated and revised, and therefore easily updated.
6 Handouts can reduce the need for note-taking.
7 Handouts and non-commercially produced leaflets can be cheap.
8 Clients and educator can work through complex information together.

Limitations

1 Professionally-produced leaflets can be expensive.
2 Mass-produced material is designed for the average consumer, and is not always suitable for everybody.
3 Commercially-produced material may contain advertising.
4 Leaflets and handouts are not durable and are easily lost.
5 Handouts demand good typing and reproducing facilities.
6 Pre-testing with consumer group is advisable.
7 Can end up as unread waste paper unless the educator actively involves the client in reading and using the material.

Posters and Charts

Uses and Advantages

1 Can raise awareness of health issues, and challenge beliefs, attitudes and behaviour.
2 Can convey information, direct people to other sources (addresses, telephone numbers, "pick up a leaflet").
3 Can be "home-made" cheaply.

Limitations

1 For small audiences only (except giant commercial posters).
2 Quickly get damaged, tatty and ignored.
3 High-quality material needs trained graphic artists and good printing equipment. This can be expensive.
4 Can be relatively expensive to buy.
5 Pre-testing with consumer group advisable.

16mm Sound Films

Uses and Advantages

1 Conveys reality (movement, sound, places, emotion) which may otherwise be inaccessible to the audience (eg. childbirth).

2 Can convey information, pose problems, demonstrate skills.
3 Can trigger discussion on attitudes and behaviour.
4 Suitable for any size of audience, including large ones.

Limitations

1 Does not permit self-pacing.
2 Films difficult and very costly to make.
3 Require an electricity supply and costly equipment (16mm projectors).
4 Equipment heavy and awkward to transport.
5 Projector requires a trained operator and can break down.
6 Films are easily damaged and expensive.
7 Darkness necessary for viewing (unless special daylight screen available) so it is difficult for the educator to observe viewers' reactions.
8 Films are often too long, with too much information and too many concepts all at once.

Videotapes and Videocassettes

Uses and Advantages

1 Conveys reality (movement, sound, places, emotion) which may otherwise be inaccessible to the audience (eg. childbirth).
2 Can convey information, pose problems, demonstrate skills.
3 Can trigger discussion on attitudes and behaviour.
4 Suitable for medium and small audiences.
5 Can be used for self-teaching and will permit self-pacing.
6 Can easily be stopped and started to permit discussion between sections. Sections can be replayed for detailed analysis.
7 Educational programmes for TV can be recorded for later use.
8 Packages including discussion notes and worksheets are being produced to link with educational TV programmes.
9 Tapes are cheaper than films, and video equipment is becoming increasingly cheap and available.
10 Little or no blackout required.
11 Equipment relatively simple to use.

Limitations

1 Electricity supply and costly equipment required.
2 Equipment can break down.
3 There are problems with the compatibility of different types of tapes, cassettes and equipment.
4 Copyright regulations for taping TV programmes are not always clear and may be restrictive.
5 Small size of screen limits size of audience.

Slides

Uses and Advantages

1 Go some way towards conveying reality.
2 Can convey information, pose problems, demonstrate skills.
3 Can trigger discussion on attitudes and behaviour.
4 Suitable for all sizes of audience including very large ones.
5 Relatively cheap and easy to produce.
6 Cheap to buy.
7 Sets of slides can be edited to suit particular audiences.
8 Can be used for self-teaching, which permits self-pacing.
9 Equipment light and easy to transport.
10 Equipment easy to use.

Limitations

1 Electricity and fairly costly equipment required.
2 Equipment can break down (but comparatively little to go wrong).
3 Needs at least partial darkness for viewing (unless special daylight screen available).

Audiotapes and Audiocassettes

Uses and Advantages

1 Especially suited to self-teaching and small groups.
2 Can be stopped and started easily to enable discussion.
3 Can convey information, pose problems, trigger discussion.
4 Good for certain skills development, eg. relaxation, exercise routines.
5 Cheap.
6 Equipment widely available.
7 Can be linked to slides to make tape/slide sets—much cheaper and easier to make than films.

Limitations

1 Good quality recording requires studio facilities.
2 Do not hold attention as well as visual material.
3 There can be problems with acoustics.

Overhead Projector Transparencies

Uses and Advantages

1 Can be used to build up information by overlaying one or more transparencies.
2 Can be prepared in advance or used to note points while teaching.
3 Educator faces audience and maintains rapport.
4 Can be used with any size of audience.
5 Cheap to buy.
6 Cheap and easy to home-produce.

7 No blackout needed.
8 Equipment relatively cheap.
9 Equipment easy to use and maintain.
10 Equipment widely available and portable overhead projectors are available.

Limitations

1 Difficult to introduce movement into visuals.
2 Ideally should have a sloping screen—otherwise the projected image is wider at the top than the bottom, and is not equally focused.
3 The lens assembly of the overhead projector can obstruct the view of the screen from some positions—careful seating arrangements are therefore necessary.
4 Requires an electricity supply.
5 Overhead projector can break down—eg. the bulb can blow.

Blackboards and Whiteboards (Wet-wipe and Dry-wipe)

Uses and Advantages

1 Good for structuring a topic and building up information in stages.
2 Good for highlighting/explaining particular points.
3 Nothing to break down!
4 No blackout needed.
5 Cheap and easily available.
6 Easily cleaned and re-used.
7 Whiteboards are easier to clean than blackboards and provide a better background for colour.
8 Permanent outlines can be drawn on whiteboards.

Limitations

1 Too small for groups of more than 25.
2 The educator has to turn her back on the audience when she writes on the board—may loose rapport.
3 Dry-wipe boards are easy to damage through incorrect cleaning—this results in shadow marking.

Flip-charts

Uses and Advantages

1 Good for "brain-storming" and for active involvement of a group in producing ideas which can be stuck up round the room for discussion.
2 Pages can be prepared in advance or used during teaching for notes and diagrams.
3 Easily portable—can be rolled or folded.
4 Can be used in rooms where there is no blackboard or whiteboard.
5 Cheap.
6 Nothing to break down.
7 No blackout needed.

Limitations

1 Too small for groups of more than 25.
2 Easily get torn and dog-eared.
3 Educator has to turn her back on the audience to write—may lose rapport.

Producing Materials

Most materials, particularly posters, leaflets, and audio-visual materials, come ready made, but some may be produced by health professionals or lay people themselves.

We have not attempted to give a comprehensive guide on how to produce materials, but we have identified some important points for making the most effective posters, displays and written materials.

Making the most of Display Materials

Posters, charts, display boards and stands.[3]

Be brief and to the point, keeping the objective firmly in mind. Do not include material which is irrelevant—it will only serve to distract from the main message.

Emphasize the key point(s) by altering the size of lettering, the style or colour. Place them just above the centre of a display, which is the point of maximum visual impact.

Use language the audience understands; explain any unfamiliar technical terms. If possible, express the message in both pictures and words. Test it out on a few people to ensure that you have no unexpected ambiguities in your message (eg. does the phrase "beating heart disease" refer to information about how to avoid getting heart disease, or is it information on a health problem known as beating-heart disease?)

Be bold. Words and pictures should be as large as possible.

Make the most of colour. It can create continuity; for example, a repetition of background colour can link a series of posters. Colour can be used to identify parts of a diagram or highlight important information. Choose colours with care, because responses to colour are emotional, eg. blue is cool, green is soothing, and because colours may be associated with certain messages, images and places, eg. red for danger, purple for funerals, white for clinical cleanliness.

Improving the display site. If all you have is a blank wall or a wall covered with a distractingly-patterned wallpaper, fix a rectangle of coloured card to the wall as a background display board. If a display board has a rough or marked surface, give it a coat of paint or a covering of coloured paper, hessian or felt.

Use the display site to best advantage. Busy corridors can only be useful sites for posters with immediate appeal and few words. More information can be conveyed in a waiting area and it may be possible to supplement displays with leaflets to take away. Ensure that writing on displays is at eye level and large enough to be read without having to move from the queue or the chair.

Be aware of lighting. Daylight is unreliable, and spotlights directed on to a display are ideal.

Making Written Materials

Instruction sheets and cards, leaflets and booklets.[4]

Always test materials on a sample of consumers. Do not *assume* that you know what they like, want or need—*ask them.*

Note the use of colour, layout and print size to improve clarity. Large print may be helpful for the elderly.

Use plain English, simple words and short sentences. Use the active tense rather than the passive tense, eg. say "change the bandage . . ." rather than "the bandage should be changed . . ."

Do a Gobbledygook readability test on your written materials.[5] The test is a rough measure of readability for adult readers based on the principle that, by and large, the combination of long sentences and polysyllabic words is harder to comprehend. It is nonetheless also important to note that many other factors which affect readability, such as sentence structure, print size and the educational background of the reader, are not taken into account.

The Gobbledygook Test

This test is based on R. Gunning's FOG (Frequency of Gobbledygook) formula and was adapted by the Plain English Campaign.

This is what you do:

— Count a 100 word sample.
— Count the number of complete sentences in the sample.
— Count the total number of words in the complete sentences.
— Divide the number of words by the number of sentences. This gives the average sentence length.
— Count the number of words with three or more syllables in the 100 words. This gives the percentage of long words in the sample.
  Numbers and symbols are counted as short words; hyphenated words are counted as two words; a syllable, for the purposes of the test, is a vowel sound. So "advised" is two syllables; "applying" is three.
— Add the average sentence length to the percentage of long words to give the test score: the higher the score, the lower the "readability".

continued on next page

continued

It is usual to do this three times to three different samples, one from the beginning of the text, one from the middle and one from near the end. These scores can then be added and divided by three to give the average score.

Tests carried out in 1980 by the National Consumer Council showed that the following publications had these scores:

Woman magazine	25
The Sun	26
Daily Mail	31
The Times	36
The Guardian	39

Exercise — The Gobbledygook Test

Do the Gobbledygook test on the following 100-word samples.

Sample 1

From now on, measures of alcohol will be stated in terms of beer, remembering that the alcohol content of all the following measures is roughly the same, so that statements made about, say, three pints of beer are also true of three doubles of spirit, or six glasses of wine, six glasses of sherry or two pints of special lager (which happens to be half as strong again as ordinary beer).

One has to consider, when trying to link intake of alcohol to the effects it has on individuals, that it is not only the amount of drink involved, but the . . .

Sample 2

We know that whooping cough vaccine works. The fact that there was so little whooping cough around when most children were immunized is one sign of how effective the vaccine is.

Remember that there are many different causes of brain damage in young children — many very much more common than whooping cough vaccine. In fact, the part played by whooping cough vaccine in causing any sort of brain damage at all is very tiny indeed.

Remember too that when doctors talk about brain damage, they do not necessarily mean severe mental handicap but usually something much less serious from which . . .

Exercise — Writing plain English

Write ''plain English'' versions of the following.
The first three are very similar to the instructions found on the packages of

continued on next page

continued

medication bought over the counter in chemist shops. The last three are very similar to passages in health education leaflets.

1. WHEEZOFF paediatric syrup is specially formulated for children. It is indicated for the relief of cough and its congestive symptoms and for the treatment of hay fever and other allergic conditions affecting the upper respiratory tract.
    Contra-indications, warnings, etc.
    Hypersensitivity to any of the active constituents. If symptoms persist consult your doctor.

2. NOTWINGE cream — directions for use.
    Apply a sufficient quantity of balm to the part affected. Massage lightly until penetration is complete.

3. SOOTHE vapour rub — how to apply.
    Rub on chest, throat and back. Then spread it thick on chest. Repeat at bedtime. Leave bedclothes loose around the neck so that the decongestant antiseptic vapours may be inhaled freely. For severe nasal catarrh, head colds, coughs and bronchitis, melt some SOOTHE in boiling water and inhale the intensified decongestant antiseptic vapours.

4. If the room has a solid fuel, oil or gas-burning appliance ensure adequate ventilation.

5. The baby lies curled up in what is called the fetal position. It lies in a bag of water and the membranes which make up this fluid-filled balloon are enclosed in the womb.

6. Vitamin B1, also called thiamin, is required for the functioning of the nervous system, digestion and metabolism. Insufficient vitamin B1 can cause anorexia and fatigue.

Presenting Statistical Information

Numbers are useful for answering questions which begin how much? how many? how long? what's the risk? But numbers can be indigestible and meaningless to lay audiences unless they are carefully presented in a visual way.[6]

The following examples of a bar chart, pictogram, histogram and pie chart show how graphics can be used to bring a pictorial dimension to dry statistics.

The *Bar Chart* in Figure 6 shows how (1) people in different parts of the world and (2) men and women have different death rates from heart disease.

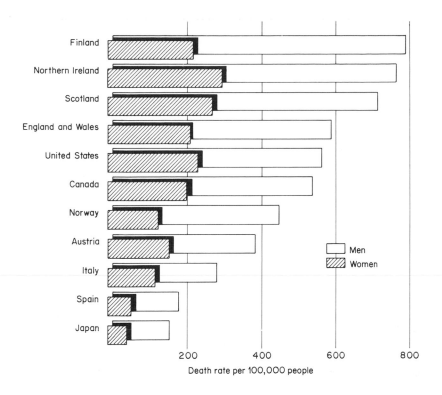

Figure 6. Death rates from coronary heart disease in different countries (35-74 year olds). (Based on figures from the World Health Organisation.)[7]

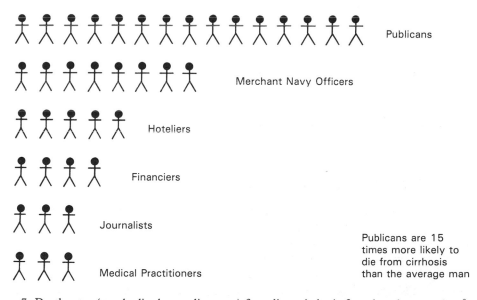

Figure 7. Death rates (standardized mortality rates) from liver cirrhosis for selected occupations[8]

The *Pictogram* (Figure 7) shows how people in different occupations have different death rates from cirrhosis of the liver. A pictogram is similar to a bar chart but uses symbols to give greater visual effect.

The *Histogram* (Figure 8) shows how the ex-smoker's risk of dying from lung cancer gradually reduces with the passage of time. A histogram is a type of graph, which uses blocks rather than a curving line to simplify the presentation of the information.

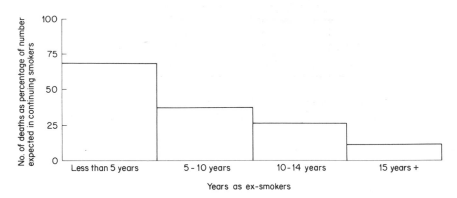

Figure 8. The relationship between the number of years as an ex-smoker and death from lung cancer (in males).[9]

The *Pie Chart* (Figure 9) shows the proportion of adults who smoke in England and Wales. A pie chart is a circle that is divided into segments (slices of the pie) so that the size of each segment is proportional to the number it represents. This example was calculated as follows:

Population of England and Wales = 41 million aged over 16 years
Number of smokers over 16 years = 15 million
41 million is represented by 360 degrees (ie. a full circle)
15 million is therefore represented by $\frac{360}{1} \times \frac{15}{41} = 131$ degrees

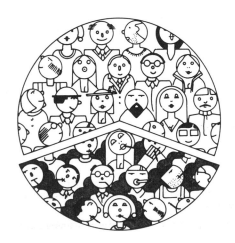

Figure 9. The proportion of adults who smoke in England and Wales.[10]

Exercise — Presenting statistical information

The following table gives statistics on the annual fatality rate from home accidents per 100,000 population in great Britain.[11]

Age	Both sexes	Male	Female
0–14	3.5	3.9	3.1
15–64	5.2	6.0	4.2
65–74	19.6	19.0	19.7
74+	106.5	88.0	115.2

What key points of information can you identify?
Draw some sketches to show how you could present this information in a visual way.

Notes, References and Further Reading

1 Useful lists of health education resources are:

Health Education Council source lists covering a range of topics, eg. food hygiene, mental health, smoking, personal relationships, ethnic minorities; these are regularly updated. 78 New Oxford Street, London WC1A 1AH

Health Education Index, published by Edsall, 124 Belgrave Road, London SW1V 2BL. This is a comprehensive listing, classified by subject, of every sort of health educational material. Each item is briefly described, and the name, address and telephone number of every supplier is included. This is regularly updated; latest edition 1984.

Health Education Resources on Women's Health, published by Paddington and North Kensington, and Victoria Health Authorities. Paddington and North Kensington Health Education Department, 304 Westbourne Grove, London W11 Tel: 01-229-9001. Victoria Health Education Department, 1a Thorndike Close, London SW10 Tel: 01-351-5495

2 Further reading on audiovisual aids:

Powell L S (1978) *A Guide to the Use of Visual Aids*. British Association for Commercial and Industrial Education

Brown J W, Lewis R B & Harcleroad F F (1977) *AV Instruction: Technology, Media and Methods*. New York: McGraw-Hill

Anderson R H (1976). *Selecting and Developing Media for Instruction*. New York: Van Nostrand Reinhold

Townsend I (1981) *A Guide to Producing Tape-slide Packages*. NHS Learning Resources Unit, 55 Bromgrove Road, Sheffield S10 2NA

Waller C (1983) *Using your Overhead Projector and Other Visual Aids*. London:

Fordigraph. Obtainable from Ofrex Ltd, Ofrex House, Stephen Street, London W1A 1EA

Wilkinson J (1979) *The Overhead Projector.* London: British Council

3 For a 22-page step-by-step guide to making health service noticeboards and displays interesting and effective, see:

Siddall S (1982) *Getting the Message Across.* Available from Bristol and Weston Health Authority Health Education Department, Central Health Clinic, Tower Hill, Bristol BS2 0JD

4 Further reading:

Adult Literacy Support Services Fund (1980) *Understanding Labels—Problems for Poor Readers.* Obtainable from Broadcasting Support Services, 252, Western Avenue, London. W3 6XY (A survey of the readability of labels on proprietary medicines, baby foods and dangerous household products.)

Ceccio J F, Ceccio C M (1982) *Effective Communication in Nursing: Theory and Practice.* New York: John Wiley (Chapter on writing readable health information for the client.)

5 The Gobbledygook Test is reproduced by kind permission of the Plain English Campaign. See also:

Cutts M & Maher C (1980) *Writing Plain English: a Guide for Writers and Designers of Official Forms, Leaflets, Letters, Labels and Agreements.* Plain English Campaign

Information and materials are available from: The Plain English Campaign, Vernon House, Whaley Bridge, Stockport SK12 7HP Telephone: 066-334541

6 For more about statistics, see:

Bayliss D (1983) Statistics for nurses 1: collection and presentation of data. *Nursing Times,* **79** (43)

Huff D (1973) *How to Lie with Statistics.* Harmondsworth: Pelican Books

7 Published in booklet:

(1982) *Beating Heart Disease.* London: Health Education Council. (Reproduced by kind permission of the Health Education Council, London.)

8 Published in:

Patton A *et al* (1981) ABC of alcohol—nature of the problem. *Br Med J,* **283,** 1319. (Reproduced by kind permission of the editor of the British Medical Journal.)

9 Lung Cancer data from:

Doll R & Peto R (1976) Mortality in relation to smoking . . . 20 years' observations in male British doctors. *Br Med J.* Pubished in the booklet, *The Facts about Smoking—What Every Nurse Should Know.* (1983) London: Health Education Council. (Reproduced by kind permission of the editor of the British Medical Journal.)

10   Published in booklet:

The Facts about Smoking—What Every Nurse Should Know. (1983) London: Health Education Council. (Reproduced by kind permission of the Health Education Council, London.)

11   Published in:

Royal Society for the Prevention of Accidents (1983). *Home and Leisure Safety for Pre-retirement Course Organisers.* (Reproduced by permission of RoSPA.)

Index